Best Practices in Nursing

Editor

ERICA L. STONE

NURSING CLINICS
OF NORTH AMERICA

www.nursing.theclinics.com

Consulting Editor
STEPHEN D. KRAU

September 2021 • Volume 56 • Number 3

ELSEVIER

1600 John F. Kennedy Boulevard • Suite 1800 • Philadelphia, Pennsylvania, 19103-2899

http://www.theclinics.com

NURSING CLINICS OF NORTH AMERICA Volume 56, Number 3
September 2021 ISSN 0029-6465, ISBN-13: 978-0-323-89726-6

Editor: Kerry Holland
Developmental Editor: Axell Ivan Jade M. Purificacion

Nursing Clinics of North America (ISSN 0029-6465) is published quarterly by Elsevier Inc., 360 Park Avenue South, New York, NY 10010-1710. Months of issue are March, June, September, and December. Periodicals postage paid at New York, NY and additional mailing offices. Subscription price per year is, $163.00 (US individuals), $669.00 (US institutions), $275.00 (international individuals), $692.00 (international institutions), $231.00 (Canadian individuals), $692.00 (Canadian institutions), $100.00 (US and Canadian students), and $135.00 (international students). To receive student/resident rate, orders must be accompanied by name of affiliated institution, date of term, and the signature of program/residency coordinator on institution letterhead. Orders will be billed at individual rate until proof of status is received. Foreign air speed delivery is included in all *Clinics* subscription prices. All prices are subject to change without notice. **POSTMASTER:** Send address changes to *Nursing Clinics*, Elsevier Health Sciences Division, Subscription Customer Service, 3251 Riverport Lane, Maryland Heights, MO 63043. **Customer Service: Telephone: 1-800-654-2452** (U.S. and Canada); **1-314-447-8871 (outside U.S. and Canada). Fax: 1-314-447-8029. E-mail: journalscustomerservice-usa@ elsevier.com** (for print support) and **journalsonlinesupport-usa@elsevier.com** (for online support).

Nursing Clinics of North America is covered in *EMBASE/Excerpta Medica, MEDLINE/PubMed (Index Medicus), Social Sciences Citation Index, Current Contents, ASCA, Cumulative Index to Nursing, RNdex Top 100,* and Allied Health Literature and International Nursing Index (INI).

Contributors

CONSULTING EDITOR

STEPHEN D. KRAU, PhD, RN, CNE
Associate Professor (Ret), Vanderbilt University School of Nursing, Nashville, Tennessee, USA

EDITOR

ERICA L. STONE, DNP, RN, FNP-C
Assistant Professor of Nursing, Vanderbilt University School of Nursing, Clinical Nurse Faculty, Nashville, Tennessee, USA

AUTHORS

KIMBERLY BAGLEY, DNP, AGPCNP-BC, AGACNP-BC, CCRN
Critical Care Nurse Practitioner, Critical Care Medicine, Duke Health, Duke Raleigh Hospital, ATTN: DRAH ICU, Raleigh, North Carolina, USA; Duke University School of Nursing, Durham, North Carolina, USA

DENISE DAWKINS, DNP, RN, CNL, CHSE
Assistant Professor, The Valley Foundation School of Nursing, San Jose State University, San Jose, California, USA

JANELLE M. DELLE, DNP, MSN, ACNP-BC
Vanderbilt University Medical Center, Nashville, Tennessee, USA

CHERYL GAZLEY, FNP-BC
Interventional Pain Center, Hendersonville, Tennessee, USA

STEPHANIE A. GEDZYK-NIEMAN, DNP, MSN, RNC-MNN
Assistant Professor, Duke University School of Nursing, Durham, North Carolina, USA

JILL HARRIS, MSN, RN
Instructor of Nursing, Vanderbilt University School of Nursing, Nashville, Tennessee, USA

TAMIKA HUDSON, DNP, APRN, FNP-C
Assistant Dean for Student Affairs & Assistant Professor in Nursing, Vanderbilt University, Nashville, Tennessee, USA

MARGARET (BETSY) BABB KENNEDY, PhD, RN, CNE
Associate Dean for Non-Tenure Track Faculty Affairs & Advancement, Professor of Nursing, Vanderbilt University School of Nursing, Nashville, Tennessee, USA

MICHELE L. KUSZAJEWSKI, DNP, RN, CHSE
Assistant Director, Center for Nursing Discovery, Duke University School of Nursing, Durham, North Carolina, USA

BRETT MORGAN, DNP, CRNA
Senior Director of Education and Practice, American Association of Nurse Anesthetists, Park Ridge, Illinois, USA

ROBINGALE PANEPINTO, DNP, FNP
Instructor of Nursing, Vanderbilt University School of Nursing, Nashville, Tennessee, USA

ABBY LUCK PARISH, DNP, AGPCNP-BC, GNP-BC, FNAP
Director of Education Innovation, Associate Professor of Nursing, Vanderbilt University School of Nursing, Nashville, Tennessee, USA

ALYSSA ROJO, MSN, RN
Nurse Research Analyst, American Association of Nurse Anesthetists, Park Ridge, Illinois, USA

LINDSEY SEVERUD, BSN, RN, CCRN
Clinical Nurse, Intensive Care Unit, Duke Raleigh Hospital, ATTN: DRAH ICU, Raleigh, North Carolina, USA

BENJAMIN SMALLHEER, PhD, RN, ACNP-BC, FNP-BC, CCRN, CNE
Associate Professor of Nursing, Duke University School of Nursing, Durham, North Carolina, USA

DENISE H. TOLA, DNP, CRNA, CHSE
Doctor of Nursing Practice Program-Nurse Anesthesia, Clinical Assistant Professor, Duke University School of Nursing, Durham, North Carolina, USA

JESSICA WELLETTE, DNP, APRN, WHNP-BC
Instructor of Nursing, Vanderbilt University School of Nursing, Nashville, Tennessee, USA

Contents

This article provides an overview of the prevalence and cause of postpartum depression in women and postnatal depression among their male partners, as well as a review of related symptoms, risk factors, and effects on children. Evidence-based screening tools, management options, and resources for patients and providers are also presented.

Delirium is a complex diagnosis characterized by inattention accompanied by either disorganized thinking or an altered level of consciousness. Delirium affects approximately 15% of older adults in the hospital. Delirium is associated with a 62% greater risk of mortality within 1 year of discharge and a significant increase in health care costs. Although the *Diagnostic and Statistical Manual of Mental Health-5* has defined delirium, its characteristics, and has recommended diagnostic tools, one of the greatest challenges has been instituting timely and effective treatments. Effective management of delirium includes nonpharmacologic and pharmacologic interventions simultaneously instituted to control agitation while exploring causation.

The opioid epidemic skyrocketed around 2017 when many pharmaceutical companies guaranteed effective pain relief with nonaddictive properties of prescription opioids. However, this has proven to be inadequate because opioid misuse has increased in the United States. These catastrophic consequences led many providers to take on a different approach to pain management in the acute and chronic setting. In the last few years, a great deal of research has focused more on a multimodal pain management approach, in hopes to decrease the rate of opioid misuse and related overdoses and help assist in putting an end to this public health crisis.

Major risks associated with inadequate discharge preparation and execution include medication errors, adverse drug events, and hospital readmissions. Nurses must develop pertinent skills to assess how the social environment impacts patients' likelihood of a safe and healthy transition back into the community as they prepare patients for discharge. Recognition and consideration of social determinants of health are critical to minimizing health disparities, enhancing health equity and supporting positive patient outcomes. Examples of strategies for enhanced discharge practices include implicit bias assessment and training, screening for food insecurity, and assessment for quality referral sources.

The registered nurse (RN) on a medical-surgical nursing unit may be the first health care professional to encounter a patient with the signs of impending respiratory failure. Importantly, the RN must recognize the signs of respiratory compromise and possess the competence and confidence to intervene without delay. Signs of respiratory deterioration, physical assessment, and respiratory laboratory studies are reviewed. Modes of oxygen therapy, basic airway management techniques, including bag mask ventilation, and use of oropharyngeal and nasopharyngeal airways are discussed. The assembly of equipment and medications frequently used for intubation are also outlined.

The insertion, use, and maintenance of peripheral and central intravenous lines are skills used by nurses in a variety of health care and hospital settings. However, patient vascular access is not without potential complications that can result in patient harm. The aim of this review is to identify and summarize nursing research standards of care, and best practices for safe management and prevention of catheter-associated bloodstream infections related to peripheral intravascular (PIV) and central intravenous (CVC) line placement. The authors focused on concepts of site selection, skin preparation and insertion, securement, and maintenance and removal criteria for PIV and CVC.

There can be multiple barriers to implementation of patient education, yet there are also multiple modalities and opportunities for engaging patients. Using frameworks and evidence from multiple disciplines can inform nursing design of patient education approaches. This article provides an introduction to educational theory and cognitive science principles such as constructivism, metacognition, deliberate practice, and cognitive load for consideration in improving the effectiveness and outcomes of patient education.

Catheter-associated urinary tract infections (CAUTI) have a high financial and human impact on patients and society at large, making CAUTI prevention strategies essential. A shift has occurred where nurses play an increased role in infection prevention. Nurses promote staff and patient education on CAUTI prevention, identification of appropriate urinary incontinence management, and implementation of bundles and patient care strategies to minimize complications from urinary incontinence management. Because they understand the severity of CAUTI and current recommendations, nurses at the bedside are in the best position to identify appropriate indications of indwelling urinary catheters and external urine collection devices for patients.

Disparities in the quality of health care for the black population have been apparent for many decades, evidenced by the high mortality and morbidity rates for the black/African American community. Major health care organizations have recognized that a culturally diverse nursing workforce is essential to improve the health of this community. Recruitment of prenursing students from the black population is vital to building a diversified workforce sensitive to the community's needs. In recent years, innovative projects have evolved to increase nurse workforce's diversity by recruiting black/African American students. This article provides background, identifies challenges, recommends solutions, and showcases successful programs.

The value of simulation-based education can be lost without a structured and purposeful guided debrief where nursing students and health care professionals are able to think critically and reflect on the experiential learning. Debriefing enhances peer-to-peer learning and aids the nursing student in formulating best practice for the next time when this encounter may occur in the clinical setting. Debriefing should be led by a trained facilitator using evidence-based methods to ensure a safe learning environment for nursing students. Debriefing is an essential learning tool that should be considered for application in the classroom, clinical, and laboratory settings.

NURSING CLINICS OF NORTH AMERICA

SERIES OF RELATED INTEREST

Critical Care Nursing Clinics of North America
https://www.ccnursing.theclinics.com/
Advances in Family Practice Nursing
http://www.advancesinfamilypracticenursing.com/

THE CLINICS ARE AVAILABLE ONLINE!
Access your subscription at:
www.theclinics.com

Preface

Best Practices in Nursing: Advocacy and Empowerment

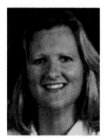

Erica L. Stone, DNP, RN, FNP-C
Editor

The nursing profession is dynamic with continual updates to its best practice standards. This issue of *Nursing Clinics of North America* provides new strategies for nurses building their patient advocacy skills while caring for vulnerable populations. Recognizing and treating postpartum depression while also simultaneously assessing and treating paternal postnatal depression is a pivotal opportunity to ensure a healthy future for our nation's children. Nurses acknowledge there are safer and more effective methods of treating both acute and chronic pain syndromes. Multimodal pain management strategies are discussed in which nurse advocacy improves patient's quality of life. There are substantial updates to safer and more effective ways for nurses to prevent, identify, and treat those suffering from delirium. This issue provides best practice standards associated with airway management and the latest strategies to reduce catheter-associated infections. Perhaps the most significant topic in this issue involves empowerment. There are updated strategies for both patient education and patient discharge to reduce the likelihood of hospital readmission. Nurses also stand at the precipice of empowering young minority students and ensuring their recruitment and retention into the nursing profession. Nurses possess the power to improve the diversity within their own profession to meet the health care needs of underserved and

Nurs Clin N Am 56 (2021) ix–x
https://doi.org/10.1016/j.cnur.2021.06.001
0029-6465/21/© 2021 Published by Elsevier Inc.

vulnerable communities. Nurses staying abreast of the best practice standards ensure a healthy future for everyone.

Erica L. Stone, DNP, RN, FNP-C
Vanderbilt University School of Nursing
461 21st Avenue South
Office #436
Nashville, TN 37240, USA

E-mail address:
Erica.l.anderson@vanderbilt.edu

Postpartum and Paternal Postnatal Depression
Identification, Risks, and Resources

Stephanie A. Gedzyk-Nieman, DNP, MSN, RNC-MNN

KEYWORDS

- Postpartum depression • Postnatal depression • Impact on children • Screening
- Treatment • Resources

KEY POINTS

- Both women and men can develop depression within 12 months of becoming parents, including by means of adoption.
- Although the exact causation of postpartum depression (PPD) in women or postnatal depression (PND) in their partners is unknown, there are several known biological, genetic, and psychosocial risk factors.
- Many professional organizations support universal screening for PPD, and some support screening for PND, but there is no universally accepted screening timeline or tool.
- Untreated PPD and PND are harmful not only to parents but potentially to their children in numerous ways.
- PPD and PND can be treated with psychosocial, psychological, and/or pharmacologic options.

INTRODUCTION

Becoming a parent brings immense joy and excitement for most women and their partners. Although it also brings great change, many women and their partners are able to adapt adequately; however, others experience serious difficulties that may include the onset of postpartum depression (PPD) in women or postnatal depression (PND) in their partners. Unlike postpartum blues (or so-called baby blues), PPD and PND are not self-limiting and require early identification and treatment in order to minimize potentially negative outcomes. This article presents a review of PPD and PND prevalence, cause, symptoms, and risk factors along with evidence-based screening tools and management options, resources for patients and providers, and information regarding the effects of untreated PPD and PND on children.

Duke University School of Nursing, 307 Trent Drive, DUMC Box 3322, Durham, NC 27710, USA
E-mail address: stephanie.gedzyknieman@duke.edu

Nurs Clin N Am 56 (2021) 325–343
https://doi.org/10.1016/j.cnur.2021.04.001
0029-6465/21/© 2021 Elsevier Inc. All rights reserved.

nursing.theclinics.com

PREVALENCE, CAUSE, AND RISK FACTORS OF POSTPARTUM DEPRESSION AND POSTNATAL DEPRESSION

Nationally in 2018, approximately 13% of women who experienced a live birth developed PPD.[1] Rates vary by state from approximately 24% in Mississippi to slightly less than 10% in Illinois,[1] and likely underrepresent the actual number of women with PPD because they reflect data based on self-reported symptoms. Women may not report symptoms of depression because they fear being stigmatized or lack understanding that such symptoms are not part of a normal postpartum recovery process.[2] In addition, women treated for PPD after their first delivery have a greater likelihood of recurrence. In a study by Rasmussen and colleagues,[3] 21% of women who required hospital care and 15% of women who required antidepressants for PPD after their first delivery were diagnosed with PPD after their second delivery.

Reported rates of PND range from 4%[4,5] to nearly 14%,[6] and, in a meta-analysis of 74 studies with more than 41,000 participants, the meta-estimate for PND was 8.4%.[7] As with PPD rates, the wide range in PND prevalence can likely be attributed to self-reported data. There is less awareness of PND compared with PPD, as well as a scarcity of related studies and a lack of consistent diagnostic and screening methods. One gap in the PND literature involves same-sex partners. All the literature regarding PND reviewed by the author for this article identified partners as male, suggesting a need for more robust attention to the prevalence and identification of PND and its effects on same-sex partners.

The cause of PPD is unknown but is likely a multifactorial, complex interaction between biological and genetic factors in conjunction with social and psychological influences, none of which occur in isolation or affect women in the same way. Guintivano and colleagues[8] examined a decade's worth of prospective studies to determine the strongest predictors of PPD. Their review failed to identify any single predictor; however, several risk factors were identified (**Fig. 1**). Risk factors with the strongest, positive associations include genetics, psychiatric history, adverse life events, and social support. Because the heritability of PPD is estimated to be between 44% and 54%, which is larger than the heritability for non–perinatal-associated depression,[9] it is imperative that health care providers inquire about both the patient's individual and familial psychiatric history.[10] Health care providers should also pay particular attention to antenatal anxiety because it has been significantly associated with PPD.[11,12]

Experiences of adverse life events can increase a patient's risk of developing PPD; these include abuse (physical, sexual, and psychological)[10,12,13] and intimate partner violence[12,14] in addition to life stressors such as financial difficulties, divorce/separation, death of a loved one, and natural disasters.[8,13,15] The importance of support during stressful life events is well documented, so lack of social support is an expected risk factor for PPD.[10,15] There is mixed evidence of PPD association with oxytocin levels, thyroid function, inflammatory markers, substance abuse, age, race, and socioeconomic status.[8]

The cause of PND, like that of PPD, is unknown and most likely multifactorial. Research has shown that fathers experience changes in brain structure, circuitry, and hormones, affecting both their response to parenthood and father-infant behaviors.[16] It is therefore likely that these biological factors, in conjunction with sociologic, economic, and psychological factors, influence the development of this disorder.

The most commonly reported risk factors for PND are provided in **Fig. 2** and are similar to those for PPD (see **Fig. 1**). One of the most frequently reported risk factors for PND is having a partner with PPD[6,17,18]; however, new evidence suggests that a

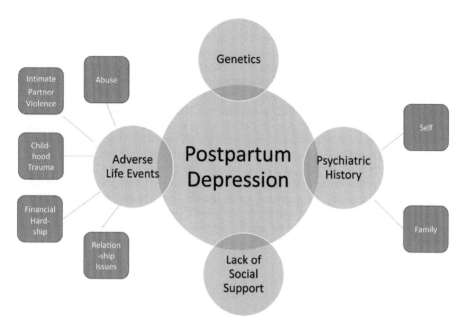

Fig. 1. Postpartum depression risk factors. (*Data From*[8] Guintivano J, Manuck T, Meltzer-Brody, S. Predictors of postpartum depression: a comprehensive review of the last decade of evidence. *Clin Obstet Gynecol.* 2018;61(3): 591–603.)

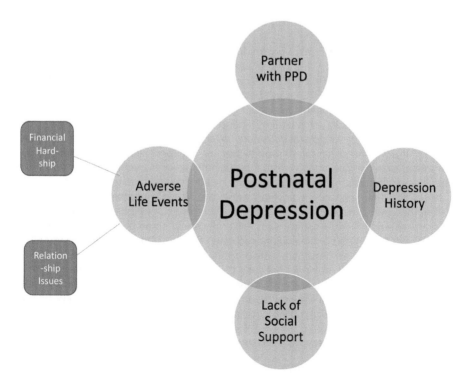

Fig. 2. Postnatal depression risk factors. (*Data from* Refs.[5,6,18–20,42])

person's risk for PND may be associated less with the partner's diagnosis of PPD than with the person's perception of the relationship with the partner after delivery. Becoming a parent is a life-altering event that causes priorities and relationships to change; if the postdelivery relationship evolves into one characterized by disconnect, discord, or a perceived decrease in support, the development of PND can be an outcome. A study by Underwood and colleagues[5] assessing postdelivery relationships between partners found no association between PPD diagnosis and PND development, but the quality of the postdelivery relationship between partners had an association with PND development. The importance of the influence of the postdelivery relationship between partners on the development of PND is similarly supported by other recent studies.[6,17–20]

In addition to considering past history of depression, health care providers should pay particular attention to any experiences of depressive symptoms reported during the partner's pregnancy, because men who develop depression during the partner's pregnancy have 7 times the risk of developing PND.[6] Factors with mixed or limited evidence of PND association include age,[6,19] smoking and poor physical health,[5] sleep quality and amount,[6] and parenting stress.[6]

SYMPTOM PRESENTATION

One reason that PPD can be missed or underreported is its similarity in presentation to a postpartum psychological experience called postpartum blues, or baby blues, considered by many to be an expected part of the postpartum recovery process. Reported rates of postpartum blues range from 39%[21] to 80%.[22] The exact cause of postpartum blues is unknown and most likely multifactorial, but, unlike PPD, postpartum blues are self-limiting, with symptoms peaking around the fifth day postpartum and resolving by the tenth day.[23] In contrast, PPD can occur at any time within 12 months after delivery, although most women experience symptoms between 2 and 12 weeks postpartum.[24]

PPD symptoms mirror those of postpartum blues, but the symptoms last longer, have greater intensity/frequency, and include lack of interest in the infant and the possibility of self-harm or infant harm (**Box 1**). *The Diagnostic and Statistical Manual of Mental Disorders* (DSM-5) describes PPD as a specifier for major depressive disorder when (1) symptom onset occurs during pregnancy or within 4 weeks after delivery and (2) the patient reports experiencing at least 5 of 9 possible symptoms for at least 2 weeks, 1 of which must be lack of interest/pleasure in activities accompanied by depressed mood.[25] If a woman or her family reports that she is experiencing thoughts of harming her infant, experiencing auditory/visual hallucinations, or experiencing delusions, she should seek immediate inpatient psychiatric care for postpartum psychosis.[23]

Like PPD, PND can occur anytime within the first 12 months after becoming a parent; however, unlike PPD, PND rates of occurrence are highest at 3 to 6 months after the event.[26] A male partner with PND may show some of the same symptoms of PPD (see **Box 1**) and can be diagnosed using the DSM-V criteria discussed earlier; however, some related behaviors, called masked male depression behaviors, may be missed by health care providers because they do not fit the traditional description of depressive symptoms. Masked male depression symptoms may include hostility and anger, isolation and social withdrawal, an increase in substance use or abuse, or risk-taking behaviors such as gambling or infidelity.[27]

POSTPARTUM DEPRESSION AND POSTNATAL DEPRESSION SCREENING

Although the anatomic and physiologic recovery from delivery usually occurs within 6 weeks, PPD can be diagnosed up to 1 year after delivery; therefore, a mother should

---

Box 1
Symptoms of postpartum blues and postpartum depression

Postpartum blues (self-resolving around day 10 postpartum):
• Depressed mood
• Crying easily or for no apparent reason
• Feeling anxious, disappointed, worthless, or overwhelmed
• Irritability or anger
• Insomnia
• Restlessness
• Fatigue
• Change in appetite
• Confusion
• Difficulty with concentration or making decisions
• Headache

PPD (requires intervention):
• Same symptoms as above, but lasting longer and with increasing intensity and frequency
• Lack of interest in the infant, family, and/or friends
• Thoughts of self-harm or infant harm

Data from Refs.[22,23,90]

---

receive initial screening for PPD at her postpartum visit followed by repeated screenings over the course of her child's first year of life. Although this maternal screening may start with the obstetric provider, it can be continued by a pediatric or family medicine provider as children are routinely seen several times during their first year of life. The NICU staff can also provide this screening for the mother of an infant who remains on their unit. Note that screening should not be limited to women who have delivered a child physically, but should include adoptive mothers because they can experience postadoption depression.[28]

While screening a mother for PPD, the health care provider can simultaneously screen the partner for PND, including adoptive fathers because they can also have PND[29]; however, because men are less likely to seek help on their own,[30] health care providers may need to find innovative ways to screen partners who do not attend postpartum or well-child visits, especially if the mother screens positive for potential PPD.

Universal screening for PPD is recommended by the American College of Obstetricians and Gynecologists[2]; the American Academy of Pediatrics[30]; the American College of Nurse Midwives[31]; the Association of Women's Health, Obstetric and Neonatal Nurses[32]; the National Perinatal Association[33]; Postpartum Support International[34]; and the US Preventive Services Task Force,[35] but only 87% of women report being asked about depression during the postpartum visit,[1] and, of these professional organizations, only the National Perinatal Association[36] and American Academy of Pediatrics[30] offer screening recommendations for PND. **Table 1** outlines assessment timelines for both PPD and PND. The recommended timing and frequency of screenings coincide with the time frame during which symptoms of PPD and PND are most likely to occur, allowing both mothers and partners several opportunities to disclose their feelings with providers, even if an appointment is missed or not attended by both individuals.

In addition to the lack of consensus on appropriate screening schedules for PPD and PND, there exists no consensus on tools to use to assess patients. In a comparative effectiveness review of 9 PPD screening tools, the Edinburgh Postnatal Depression Scale (EPDS) was used by the largest number of studies; however, based on the

Table 1
Postpartum depression and postnatal depression assessment timeline recommendations

	Prenatally and Immediate Postpartum Period	1-mo Well-baby Visit	6 wk Postpartum	2-mo Well-baby Visit	4-mo Well-baby Visit	6-mo Well-baby Visit	9-mo Well-baby Visit	12-mo Well-baby Visit
Mother	X[a]	X	X[a]	X[a]	X[a]	X[a]	X	X
Partner	—	—	—	X[a]	X[a]	X[a]	X	X

[a] Minimum recommendations.
Data from Refs.[30,33,34,36]

evidence, a recommendation could not be made for use of the EPDS rather than other tools.[37] Most instruments used to screen for depression emphasize traditional symptoms of depression, which are aligned with female-specific symptoms of depression more than with male-specific symptoms, adding another layer of difficulty to screening men for PND.[38,39] Note that tools only screen for PPD or PND. A positive screen indicates that the patient should be referred to a mental health professional for additional assessment, diagnosis, and treatment. Some of the most frequently used tools are listed in **Table 2** and are briefly described here.

The Edinburgh Postnatal Depression Scale

The EPDS is one of the most widely used screening tools. It is recommended for PPD screening by Postpartum Support International[34] and the US Preventive Services Taskforce,[35] and the American Academy of Pediatrics recommends its use for both PPD and PND screening.[30] The benefits of this tool include its length and lack of cost, as well as its inclusion of items addressing anxiety, depressive symptoms, and suicidal ideation. Patients respond to 10 items with a score from 0 to 3 based on how they have felt during the past 7 days. The total possible score is 30, and a total score of 9 or greater, or a single score of 1 or higher on item number 10 (which addresses suicidal thoughts), warrants referral to a mental health professional.[40,41] However, when translated into different languages and used with women from different cultural groups, the specificity and sensitivity of the tool vary widely, indicating that it may lack effectiveness among women from diverse groups.[41]

Although this tool is deemed statistically reliable in identifying PND, the scoring recommendations for men lack uniformity. Some researchers recommend using a lower cutoff score (5–6) because men tend to identify only 7 items on the scale as potentially problematic (especially the item regarding crying)[42]; other researchers[43,44] recommend using a score of 10 or greater. Regardless of the total score, a response of 1 or greater on item number 10 indicates the need to be seen by a mental health professional.

The Beck Depression Inventory II

This widely used depression screening tool was revised in 1996 to align with the DSM-IV criteria for depression and is available in many languages. Patients are asked to review 21 items and select the statement that best describes their feelings during the past 2 weeks. Each item has a possible score of 0 to 3 for a total possible score of 63. Scores of 14 or greater may indicate depression and warrant a referral to a mental health provider.[45,46] Despite the alignment of the Beck Depression Inventory II (BDI-II)

Table 2
Postpartum depression and postnatal depression screening tools

	Items (N)	Subscales (N)	Languages Available Beyond English	Reliability[c]	Tool Links
Edinburgh Postnatal Depression Scale[a]	10	None	19	0.87 0.81[a]	https://www.mcpapformoms.org/Docs/Edinburgh%2520Depression%25205cale%2520Translated%2520Government%2520of%2520Western%2520Australia%2520Department%2520of%2520Health.pdf
Edinburgh Gotland Depression Scale[b]	12	None	English	0.91	See Psouni et al[51]
Beck Depression Inventory II	21	None	Spanish	0.83–0.95	https://www.pearsonassessments.com/store/usassessments/en/Store/Professional-Assessments/Personality-%2526-Biopsychosocial/Beck-Depression-Inventory-II/p/100000159.html
Center for Epidemiologic Studies Depression Scale	20	None	13	0.85	https://cesd-r.com/
Gotland Scale for Male Depression[b]	13	2	Swedish	0.86–0.88 (Swedish)	See Zierau et al[50]
Patient Health Questionnaire 9[a]	9	None	Abundant	0.86	https://www.phqscreeners.com/
Postpartum Depression Screening Scale	35	7	Italian Spanish	Subscale scores range 0.80–0.91	https://www.wpspublish.com/pdss-postpartum-depression-screening-scale

[a] Recommended for PND screening as well.
[b] PND screening only.
[c] Data reported for English version of the tool unless otherwise noted.
Data from Refs.[2,17,33,40,41,43,48,50,51,87–89]

with the DSM-IV criteria for depression, it may require modifications to screen for PPD. Logistic regression conducted by Conradt and colleagues[45] revealed that using the total score on the BDI-II may overestimate PPD risk; the investigators suggest focusing instead on 4 items that most often predict PPD (changes in appetite, pessimism, loss of interest, and sadness).

The Patient Health Questionnaire 9

This free 9-question tool aligns with the DSM-V criteria for depression but, unlike other tools available, does not include items to assess for anxiety. It has been recommended by the American Academy of Pediatrics[30] and Postpartum Support International[34] for PPD screening, and by Postpartum Support International[34] for PND screening. Scores range from 0 to 3 for each of the 9 items, for a total possible score of 27. It is recommended that both men and women with a score of 10 or greater be referred to a mental health professional.[47]

The Postpartum Depression Screening Scale and the Center for Epidemiologic Studies Depression Scales

The Postpartum Depression Screening Scale (PDSS) ranks second to the EPDS for frequency of use in screening for PPD.[37] It requires purchase and is lengthier than other tools; however, it includes 7 subscales covering dimensions of PPD that may be helpful for a more comprehensive screening. The patient is asked to answer 35 items on a 5-point Likert scale based on how they have felt during the past 2 weeks. Total scores can range from 35 to 175, with a recommended score of 60 or greater indicating need for referral to a mental health provider.[48] Unlike the EPDS, the PDSS has been used to screen for PPD only.

The CESD-R, a free 20-item tool used to screen for PPD only, is available in multiple languages. Patients are asked to rate the frequency with which they experience symptoms on a scale ranging from 0 (not at all or <1 day) to 4 (nearly every day for 2 weeks). Total scores can range from 0 to 60, with a recommended score of 16 or greater warranting further assessments.[49]

The Gotland Scale for Male Depression and the Edinburgh Gotland Depression Scale

As many screening tools for depression focus heavily on female-specific depression symptoms,[38,39] the 13-item Gotland Scale for Male Depression (GSMD) was developed to address the challenge of identifying depression in men. Men are asked to rank each behavior-based item on a 4-point Likert scale with scores ranging from 0 to 3 according to how the specified behavior has changed (if at all) over the past month. The total possible score range is 0 to 39, with a score of 13 or greater warranting further evaluation.[50] A study by Carlberg and colleagues[43] evaluated the effectiveness of the EPDS compared with the GSMD in capturing possible PND. In many cases, possible depression was detected in participants by 1 of the 2 instruments alone, but not by both, supporting previous evidence that neither scale is ideal and that they likely assess different aspects of depression.

Psouni and colleagues[51] pooled the items on the EPDS and GSMD, conducted a factor analysis, and devised the Edinburgh Gotland Depression Scale, on which a patient is asked to rate 12 items on a 4-point Likert scale based on how they have felt over the past 2 weeks. Possible total scores range from 0 to 36, with a score of 12 or greater, or of 1 or greater on the single item regarding thoughts of self-harm, warranting further evaluation.[51] The scarcity of published studies regarding use of this tool for assessment of PND is an important consideration.

EFFECT OF POSTPARTUM DEPRESSION/POSTNATAL DEPRESSION ON CHILDREN

Screening for and treatment of PPD/PND are important for new parents but also for their children. Children of parents with depression can develop negative health outcomes caused by exposure to toxic stress. Toxic stress results from the "strong, frequent, or prolonged activation of the body's stress response systems in the absence of the buffering protection of a supportive, adult relationship."[52(p236)] PPD has been identified as a source of toxic stress in children because these mothers are unable to provide for them fully or to foster a sufficiently supportive relationship to mitigate their stress response. In infants, exposure to toxic stress causes disruptions in the brain's neurobiology and neurocircuitry, with negative health consequences. Lebel and colleagues[53] conducted MRI scans on preschool-aged children to examine whether changes in their brain structure were associated with their mothers' PPD scores at 2 to 3 months after delivery. The PPD scores were found to be negatively correlated with the child's right cortical thickness and white matter diffusivity. These brain regions are thought to play a role in executive functioning, controlling inhibitions, attention span, anxiety, and depression.

It is estimated that children born to mothers diagnosed with PPD are 2 to 3 times more likely to experience behavioral, social, and/or emotional difficulties later in life.[54–56] These difficulties can develop as early as 12 months of age but may not be revealed until the child enters the educational system. Slomian and colleagues[57] conducted a systematic review of 67 studies regarding the impact of PPD on infants and found a vast amount of evidence supporting negative effects of maternal PPD on infant cognitive and language development, behaviors, and overall health concerns. Negative behaviors seen in children of mothers with PPD include hyperactivity[58]; anxiety and separation distress[59]; depression[58,60]; sensory sensitivity[59]; and impulsivity, aggression, and difficulty expressing empathy.[59]

In addition to the social-emotional effects of PPD on children, there are cognitive effects. Children of mothers with PPD have lower overall academic performance scores[61,62] and lower mathematics scores.[58] These children also have approximately a 7-point reduction in IQ scores compared with children whose mothers were never depressed,[63] and they are more likely to require special education services, especially if the mother belongs to a low socioeconomic group.[64]

PPD further hurts children in that it impairs the maternal-infant bonding process and negatively affects the quality of that bond. In 1 systematic review regarding prenatal and postpartum maternal-infant bonding quality, it was revealed that 28 of 29 studies focused on PPD had found moderate to strong negative correlations between PPD and maternal-infant bonding.[65] Impaired bonding can decrease a mother's sensitivity/attention to or accurate assessment of infant cues, thus jeopardizing the child's health and safety. One study found that children of mothers who had PPD at 12 and 24 months after delivery had higher occurrences of injuries (eg, burns, falls, cuts) compared with children of mothers who did not have PPD.[66] Another study found that such children also had higher rates of acute illnesses than children of women without PPD.[67]

There is evidence that impaired bonding can negatively affect the relationship the mother has with her child when that child becomes an adult. Myers and Johns[68] found that mothers who had PPD had a less positive perception of the quality of the relationship with that adult child than mothers who had not had PPD. Also, the more severe the mother's symptoms of PPD had been, the lower her perceived quality of the mother-adult child relationship. Findings showed that the effects of PPD were intergenerational; grandmothers who had been diagnosed with PPD reported having a lesser level of emotional closeness with the children of the child whose delivery had been followed by PPD.

Lack of identification and treatment of PND in fathers can also contribute to negative health outcomes for the child. A father can serve as a buffer to toxic stress when the mother cannot; however, if the father also has depression, his ability to serve in this role is diminished, leaving the child even more susceptible to the negative effects of toxic stress. Negative behaviors seen in children of fathers with PND include anxiety and separation distress,[59] sensory sensitivity,[59] and difficulty with empathy,[59] as well as depression, particularly in female children[69] or children of a father with minimal education.[60]

Similar to the effects of a mother's experience of PPD, a father's experience of PND can negatively influence the child's academic performance[61] as well as father-child attachment and safety. Fathers with PND have less patience with their infants, obtain less enjoyment from interacting with their infants, and show less affection toward their infants.[70] Because these behaviors are necessary for parent-infant attachment to occur, an infant who is deprived of them is at risk for impaired social development and injury. One study found that infants whose fathers had PND 2 months after their birth were more likely to be maltreated or have their safety jeopardized,[71] possibly because of the fathers' decreased sensitivity/attention to or accurate assessment of infant cues.

MANAGEMENT OF POSTPARTUM DEPRESSION/POSTNATAL DEPRESSION

Once a diagnosis of PPD is made, there are various levels of care that can be used to manage this disease. Once initiated, therapy for PPD has been shown to be fairly effective. One year after initiating treatment (either via pharmacotherapy or other supportive measures), only 28% of patients still required treatment, and, after 4 years, only 5% were still in treatment.[3]

Stewart and Vigod[72] propose a stepped care approach to PPD treatment that begins with supportive interventions with the option to add additional interventions as necessary based on patient response and symptoms (**Fig. 3**). The initial intervention includes supportive psychosocial and self-care strategies (eg, promotion of sleep, exercise, stress management). A meta-analysis has indicated that improved infant sleep has a small positive effect on mother's mood,[73] and light-to-moderate exercise has been shown to be an effective adjunctive therapy for reducing PPD symptoms.[74] Exercise (in various forms) has also been found to improve patients' perceived quality of life and to reduce fatigue.[75] Psychosocial support can be provided by a health care professional or a peer support person. Peer support programs for PPD via telephone, in the home, or in a group setting have resulted in significant reductions in PPD symptoms and high patient satisfaction.[76]

If initial interventions prove unsuccessful, providers can add psychological therapies, such as cognitive behavior therapy (CBT) or interpersonal therapy (IPT), and/or an antidepressant to the regimen. CBT is the most used form of psychological therapy found in PPD literature.[77,78] Meta-analysis of 10 trials examining the efficacy of CBT and IPT in treating PPD showed a significant improvement in PPD symptoms, both in the immediate period after treatment and 6 months later, as well as a reduction in stress and anxiety.[78] Although CBT is the most commonly used form of psychological therapy, no difference was found in improvement of symptoms resulting from CBT compared with IPT, or in results associated with individual therapy compared with therapy provided in a group setting. Similar findings were reported by O'Connor and colleagues[77] in their systematic review. Note that, in the meta-analysis, trained

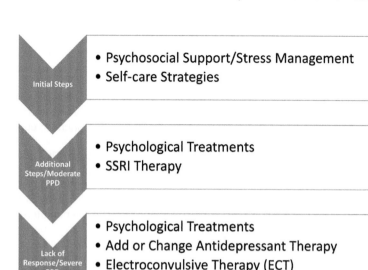

Fig. 3. Postpartum depression management. (*Data From*[72] Stewart DE, Vigod SN. Postpartum depression: pathophysiology, treatment, and emerging therapeutics. *Annu Rev Med.* 2019;70:183-196.)

community nurses provided most of the CBT or IPT, which shows the importance of nurses to interdisciplinary team care for these patients.

In the PPD literature, selective serotonin reuptake inhibitors (SSRIs) are the most commonly prescribed antidepressants,[72] with sertraline being the most frequently studied SSRI.[79] A systematic review[80] and a Cochrane Review with meta-analysis[81] both found that patients using SSRIs had greater reduction of PPD symptoms and remission compared with placebo. If all of the interventions mentioned earlier are ineffective, or if the patient has severe symptoms, electroconvulsive therapy can be considered. Regardless of proposed interventions, it is important to include the patient and allow her to choose the options she considers most feasible given her daily schedule, finances, childcare needs, and/or breastfeeding needs.

Recently a new treatment of PPD became available. In March 2019, Zulresso (brexanolone) became the first drug approved specifically for the treatment of PPD.[82] Although its mechanism of action is not completely understood, it is thought that Zulresso serves as a gamma-aminobutyric acid A (GABAA) receptor positive modulator that improves the response to naturally occurring GABA in the body.[83] Levels of the naturally occurring GABAA positive modulator allopregnanolone decrease significantly after delivery, and this is thought to be a possible factor in the development of PPD.[84]

Because of the risk of excessive sedation or sudden loss of consciousness, Zulresso can only be administered to patients via a Risk Evaluation and Mitigation Strategy program. This program includes (1) administering the drug in a certified health care facility to allow the monitoring necessary to maintain patient safety; (2) not allowing the patient to be left alone with her child/children; and (3) administering the drug as a continuous, titrated intravenous infusion over a total of 60 hours (2.5 days).

The early data regarding Zulresso's effectiveness are promising. In 2 double-blind, randomized, placebo-controlled studies with participants with moderate or severe PPD, participants who received Zulresso had greater improvement in symptoms both at the end of the infusion and 30 days postinfusion.[84] Although rapid onset of improvement is an impressive benefit of using this drug, data to determine its long-term efficacy beyond 30 days postinfusion are unavailable.[84] These data are needed for comparison with the long-term efficacy of oral antidepressants.

Zulresso's cost could also be a barrier to equitable and widespread use. Its list price is more than $7000 per vial, with a projected cost of $34,000 for the 4.5 vials needed for treatment,[85] and this does not include facility charges for the 60+ hours of care required for administration.

Literature on the management of PND is minimal. The author found only 1 RCT that examined the effects of group lifestyle-based training (sleep, physical activity, nutrition, sexual health, and self-image) on paternal depression and anxiety[86]; after completing the training, participants experienced a significant decrease in both outcomes compared with the control group. Additional research needs to be conducted in order to meet the specialized needs of fathers with PND.

Box 2
Resources for postpartum depression and postnatal depression

- American Academy of Pediatrics: https://www.healthychildren.org/English/ages-stages/prenatal/Pages/Depression-and-Anxiety-During-Pregnancy-and-After-Birth-FAQs.aspx
- American Academy of Pediatrics (Paternal Postpartum Depression): https://www.healthychildren.org/English/ages-stages/prenatal/delivery-beyond/Pages/Dads-Can-Get-Postpartum-Depression-Too.aspx
- American College of Obstetricians and Gynecologists: https://www.acog.org/patient-resources/faqs/labor-delivery-and-postpartum-care/postpartum-depression
- American Psychological Association: https://www.apa.org/pi/women/resources/reports/postpartum-depression
- Centers for Disease Control and Prevention: https://www.cdc.gov/reproductivehealth/depression/index.htm
- March of Dimes: https://www.marchofdimes.org/pregnancy/postpartum-depression.aspx
- Massachusetts General Hospital Center for Women's Mental Health: https://womensmentalhealth.org/
- Medline Plus: https://medlineplus.gov/postpartumdepression.html
- National Institutes of Health National Child & Maternal Health Education Program: https://www.nichd.nih.gov/ncmhep/initiatives/moms-mental-health-matters/moms
- National Institute of Mental Health: https://www.nimh.nih.gov/health/publications/perinatal-depression/index.shtml
- National Perinatal Association: http://www.nationalperinatal.org/mental_health
- PPD (maternal and paternal depression): https://www.postpartumdepression.org/
- Postpartum Men: http://postpartummen.com/
- Postpartum Progress: https://postpartumprogress.com
- Postpartum Support International: https://www.postpartum.net/
- US Preventive Services Taskforce: https://www.uspreventiveservicestaskforce.org/uspstf/recommendation/perinatal-depression-preventive-interventions
- World Health Organization: https://www.who.int/mental_health/maternal-child/maternal_mental_health/en/

SUMMARY

Both women and men can experience depression after the birth or adoption of a child. The prevalence of this type of depression is difficult to determine because it (1) is based on self-reported data, (2) can be misdiagnosed as the baby blues, and (3) may present in men with behaviors not typically identified as depression symptoms. Its exact cause is unknown but is most likely influenced by a combination of biological, genetic, social, and psychological factors.

Although numerous professional organizations support universal screening for depression after the birth of a child, there is a lack of consensus regarding how often these screenings should occur and what tools should be used; this ambiguity is more pronounced regarding screening of men. Of the several tools presented in this article, the EPDS is most commonly used to screen women and has been used to screen men; however, all of the tools presented in this article have strengths and weaknesses and should be examined closely before their implementation.

Exposure to a depressed parent can cause negative health, psychological, neurologic, academic, emotional, behavioral, and social short-term and long-term outcomes for children; therefore, treatment of this type of depression is important not only for parents and their partners but for their children. Treatment options for PPD include psychosocial and self-care activities, CBT or IPT, antidepressants, and, for serious cases, electroconvulsive therapy. A new pharmacotherapy, Zulresso (brexanolone), is available as the first drug specifically approved to treat PPD; however, its availability is limited because of cost and administration requirements. The literature on treating PND is scarce, but positive outcomes have been reported for the use of lifestyle-based training.

CLINICS CARE POINTS

- If PPD or PND is suspected, discuss it with the patients and do not avoid asking pointed questions.
- Share the facts about PPD and PND. Reassure the patients that they are not alone and are not to blame for their feelings.
- Inform the patient and her partner of the importance of screening and supporting fathers and partners.
- When screening for PPD or PND, let the patient know that such screening is becoming universal and that they are receiving standard, best-practice care, not being singled out.
- Inform the patients that PPD and PND are treatable, and provide them with appropriate referrals and resources (**Box 2**).

DISCLOSURE

The author has nothing to disclose and no conflicts of interest.

REFERENCES

1. Bauman BL, Ko JY, Cox S, et al. Postpartum depressive symptoms and provider discussions about perinatal depression — United States, 2018. MMWR Morb Mortal Wkly Rep 2020;69(19):575–81.
2. American College of Obstetricians and Gynecologists. Committee opinion no. 757: screening for perinatal depression. Obstet Gynecol 2018;132(5):e208–12.

3. Rasmussen M-LH, Strøm M, Wohlfahrt J, et al. Risk, treatment duration, and recurrence risk of postpartum affective disorder in women with no prior psychiatric history: a population-based cohort study. PLoS Med 2017;14(9): e1002392–405.

4. Cheng ER, Downs SM, Carroll AE. Prevalence of depression among fathers at the pediatric well-child care visit. JAMA Pediatr 2018;172(9):882–3.

5. Underwood L, Waldie KE, Peterson E, et al. Paternal depression symptoms during pregnancy and after childbirth among participants in the Growing Up in New Zealand Study. JAMA Psychiatry 2017;74(4):360–9.

6. Da Costa D, Danieli C, Abrahamowicz M, et al. A prospective study of postnatal depressive symptoms and associated risk factors in first-time fathers. J Affect Disord 2019;249:371–7.

7. Cameron EE, Sedov ID, Tomfohr-Madsen LM. Prevalence of paternal depression in pregnancy and the postpartum: an updated meta-analysis. J Affect Disord 2016;206:189–203.

8. Guintivano J, Manuck T, Meltzer-Brody S. Predictors of postpartum depression: a comprehensive review of the last decade of evidence. Clin Obstet Gynecol 2018; 61(3):591–603.

9. Viktorin A, Meltzer-Brody S, Kuja-Halkola R, et al. Heritability of perinatal depression and genetic overlap with nonperinatal depression. Am J Psychiatry 2016; 173(2):158–65.

10. Bayrampour H, Tomfohr L, Tough S. Trajectories of perinatal depressive and anxiety symptoms in a community cohort. J Clin Psychiatry 2016;77(11):1467–73.

11. Grigoriadis S, Graves L, Peer M, et al. A systematic review and meta-analysis of the effects of antenatal anxiety on postpartum outcomes. Arch Womens Ment Health 2019;22(5):543–56.

12. Khanlari S, Eastwood J, Barnett B, et al. Psychosocial and obstetric determinants of women signalling distress during Edinburgh Postnatal Depression Scale (EPDS) screening in Sydney, Australia. BMC Pregnancy Childbirth 2019; 19(1):407.

13. Sidebottom AC, Hellerstedt WL, Harrison PA, et al. An examination of prenatal and postpartum depressive symptoms among women served by urban community health centers. Arch Womens Ment Health 2014;17(1):27–40.

14. Chaves K, Eastwood J, Ogbo FA, et al. Intimate partner violence identified through routine antenatal screening and maternal and perinatal health outcomes. BMC Pregnancy Childbirth 2019;19(1):357–67.

15. Leonard KS, Evans MB, Kjerulff KH, et al. Postpartum perceived stress explains the association between perceived social support and depressive symptoms. Womens Health Issues 2020;30(4):231–9.

16. Swain JE, Dayton CJ, Kim P, et al. Progress on the paternal brain: theory, animal models, human brain research, and mental health implications. Infant Ment Health J 2014;35(5):394–408.

17. Matthey S, Barnett B, Ungerer J, et al. Paternal and maternal depressed mood during the transition to parenthood. J Affect Disord 2000;60(2):75–85.

18. Nath S, Psychogiou L, Kuyken W, et al. The prevalence of depressive symptoms among fathers and associated risk factors during the first seven years of their child's life: findings from the Millennium Cohort Study. BMC Public Health 2016; 16:509.

19. Gray PB, Reece J-A, Coore-Desai C, et al. Patterns and predictors of depressive symptoms among Jamaican fathers of newborns. Soc Psychiatry Psychiatr Epidemiol 2018;53(10):1063–70.

20. Shaheen NA, AlAtiq Y, Thomas A, et al. Paternal postnatal depression among fathers of newborn in Saudi Arabia. Am J Mens Health 2019;13(1):1–12.

21. Rezaie-Keikhaie K, Arbabshastan ME, Rafiemanesh H, et al. Systematic review and meta-analysis of the prevalence of the maternity blues in the postpartum period. J Obstet Gynecol Neonatal Nurs 2020;49(2):127–36.

22. March of Dimes. Baby blues after pregnancy. 2017. Available at: https://www.marchofdimes.org/pregnancy/baby-blues-after-pregnancy.aspx. Accessed August 26, 2020.

23. Lowdermilk DL, Perry SE, Cashion K, et al. Maternity and women's health care. 12th edition. Elsevier; 2020.

24. Stowe ZN, Hostetter AL, Newport DJ. The onset of postpartum depression: implications for clinical screening in obstetrical and primary care. Am J Obstet Gynecol 2005;192(2):522–6.

25. American Psychiatric Association. Diagnostic and statistical manual of mental disorders. 5th edition. American Psychiatric Association; 2013. https://doi.org/10.1176/appi.books.9780890425596.

26. Paulson JF, Bazemore SD. Prenatal and postpartum depression in fathers and its association with maternal depression: a meta-analysis. JAMA 2010;303(19):1961–9.

27. Freitas CJ, Williams-Reade J, Distelberg B, et al. Paternal depression during pregnancy and postpartum: an international Delphi study. J Affect Disord 2016;202:128–36.

28. Foli KJ, South SC, Lim E, et al. Maternal postadoption depression, unmet expectations, and personality traits. J Am Psychiatr Nurses Assoc 2012;18(5):267–77.

29. Foli KJ, South SC, Lim E, et al. Depression in adoptive fathers: an exploratory mixed methods study. Psychol Men Masculinity 2013;14(4):411–22.

30. Earls MF, Yogman MW, Mattson G, et al. American Academy of Pediatrics Committee on Psychosocial Aspects of Child and Family Health. Incorporating recognition and management of perinatal depression into pediatric practice. Pediatrics 2019;143(1):e20183259.

31. American College of Nurse Midwives. Position statement: depression in women. 2013. Available at: https://www.midwife.org/acnm/files/ACNMLibraryData/UPLOADFILENAME/000000000061/Depression%2520in%2520Women%2520May%25202013.pdf. Accessed October 1, 2020.

32. Association of Women's Health, Obstetric and Neonatal Nurses. AWHONN position statement: mood and anxiety disorders in pregnant and postpartum women. J Obstet Gynecol Neonatal Nurs 2015;44(5):687–9.

33. Willis TN, Brook Chavis L, Saxton SN, et al. National Perinatal Association Position Statement 2018 perinatal mood and anxiety disorders. 2018. Available at: http://www.nationalperinatal.org/resources/Documents/Position%2520Papers/2018%2520Position%2520Statement%2520PMADs_NPA.pdf. Accessed October 1, 2020.

34. Postpartum Support International. Screening recommendations. Available at: https://www.postpartum.net/professionals/screening/. Accessed August 23, 2020.

35. Siu AL, US Preventative Services Taskforce. Screening for depression in adults: US Preventive Services Task Force recommendation statement. JAMA 2016;315(4):380–7.

36. Hynan MT, Mounts KO. Depression screening for new fathers. 2013. Available at: http://www.nationalperinatal.org/resources/Documents/Position%2520Papers/

Depression%2520Screening%2520for%2520New%2520Fathers%2520pdf.pdf. Accessed October 1, 2020.

37. Myers ER, Aubuchon-Endsley N, Bastian LA, et al. Efficacy and safety of screening for postpartum depression. Agency for Healthcare Research and Quality (US); 2013. Available at: http://www.ncbi.nlm.nih.gov/books/NBK137724/. Accessed October 8, 2020.

38. Albicker J, Hölzel LP, Bengel J, et al. Prevalence, symptomatology, risk factors and healthcare services utilization regarding paternal depression in Germany: study protocol of a controlled cross-sectional epidemiological study. BMC Psychiatry 2019;19(1):289.

39. O'Brien AP, McNeil KA, Fletcher R, et al. New fathers' perinatal depression and anxiety—treatment options: an integrative review. Am J Mens Health 2017; 11(4):863–76.

40. Cox JL, Holden JM, Sagovsky R. Detection of postnatal depression: development of the 10-item Edinburgh Postnatal Depression Scale. Br J Psychiatry 1987; 150(6):782–6.

41. Gibson J, McKenzie-McHarg K, Shakespeare J, et al. A systematic review of studies validating the Edinburgh Postnatal Depression Scale in antepartum and postpartum women. Acta Psychiatr Scand 2009;119(5):350–64.

42. Matthey S, Barnett B, Kavanagh DJ, et al. Validation of the Edinburgh Postnatal Depression Scale for men, and comparison of item endorsement with their partners. J Affect Disord 2001;64(2):175–84.

43. Carlberg M, Edhborg M, Lindberg L. Paternal perinatal depression assessed by the Edinburgh Postnatal Depression Scale and the Gotland Male Depression Scale: prevalence and possible risk factors. Am J Mens Health 2018;12(4):720–9.

44. Edmondson OJH, Psychogiou L, Vlachos H, et al. Depression in fathers in the postnatal period: assessment of the Edinburgh Postnatal Depression Scale as a screening measure. J Affect Disord 2010;125(1):365–8.

45. Conradt E, Manian N, Bornstein MH. Screening for depression in the postpartum using the Beck Depression Inventory-II: what logistic regression reveals. J Reprod Infant Psychol 2012;30(5):427–35.

46. Ghosh Ippen C, Wong C. Beck depression inventory. 2nd edition. The National Child Traumatic Stress Network; 2014. Available at: https://www.nctsn.org/measures/beck-depression-inventory-second-edition. Accessed October 30, 2020.

47. Instructions for Patient Health Questionnaire (PHQ) and GAD-7 Measures. Available at: https://www.phqscreeners.com/images/sites/g/files/g10016261/f/201412/instructions.pdf. Accessed October 1, 2020.

48. Beck CT, Gable RK. Further validation of the postpartum depression screening scale. Nurs Res 2001;50(3):155–64.

49. CESD-R: Center for Epidemiologic Studies Depression Scale Revised Online Depression Assessment. CESD-R: Center for Epidemiologic Studies Depression Scale Revised Online Depression Assessment. Available at: https://cesd-r.com/. Accessed October 30, 2020.

50. Zierau F, Bille A, Rutz W, et al. The Gotland Male Depression Scale: a validity study in patients with alcohol use disorder. Nord J Psychiatry 2002;56(4):265–71.

51. Psouni E, Agebjörn J, Linder H. Symptoms of depression in Swedish fathers in the postnatal period and development of a screening tool. Scand J Psychol 2017;58(6):485–96.

52. Shonkoff JP, Garner AS, The Committee on Psychosocial Aspects of Child and Family Health, Committee on Early Childhood, Adoption, and Dependent Care,

Section on Developmental and Behavioral Pediatrics. The lifelong effects of early childhood adversity and toxic stress. Pediatrics 2012;129(1):e232–46.

53. Lebel C, Walton M, Letourneau N, et al. Prepartum and postpartum maternal depressive symptoms are related to children's brain structure in preschool. Biol Psychiatry 2016;80(11):859–68.

54. Giallo R, Woolhouse H, Gartland D, et al. The emotional–behavioural functioning of children exposed to maternal depressive symptoms across pregnancy and early childhood: a prospective Australian pregnancy cohort study. Eur Child Adolesc Psychiatry 2015;24(10):1233–44.

55. Junge C, Garthus-Niegel S, Slinning K, et al. The impact of perinatal depression on children's social-emotional development: a longitudinal study. Matern Child Health J 2017;21(3):607–15.

56. Woolhouse H, Gartland D, Mensah F, et al. Maternal depression from pregnancy to 4 years postpartum and emotional/behavioural difficulties in children: results from a prospective pregnancy cohort study. Arch Womens Ment Health 2016; 19(1):141–51.

57. Slomian J, Honvo G, Emonts P, et al. Consequences of maternal postpartum depression: a systematic review of maternal and infant outcomes. Womens Health (Lond) 2019;15. https://doi.org/10.1177/1745506519844044.

58. Netsi E, Pearson RM, Murray L, et al. Association of persistent and severe postnatal depression with child outcomes. JAMA Psychiatry 2018;75(3):247.

59. Fredriksen E, von Soest T, Smith L, et al. Parenting stress plays a mediating role in the prediction of early child development from both parents' perinatal depressive symptoms. J Abnorm Child Psychol 2019;47(1):149–64.

60. Pearson RM, Evans J, Kounali D, et al. Maternal depression during pregnancy and the postnatal period: risks and possible mechanisms for offspring depression at age 18 years. JAMA Psychiatry 2013;70(12):1312–9.

61. Psychogiou L, Russell G, Owens M. Parents' postnatal depressive symptoms and their children's academic attainment at 16 years: pathways of risk transmission. Br J Psychol 2020;111(1):1–16.

62. Shen H, Magnusson C, Rai D, et al. Associations of parental depression with child school performance at age 16 years in Sweden. JAMA Psychiatry 2016;73(3): 239–46.

63. van der Waerden J, Bernard JY, Agostini MD, et al. Persistent maternal depressive symptoms trajectories influence children's IQ: the EDEN mother–child cohort. Depress Anxiety 2017;34(2):105–17.

64. Ride J. Is socioeconomic inequality in postnatal depression an early-life root of disadvantage for children? Eur J Health Econ 2019;20(7):1013–27.

65. Tichelman E, Westerneng M, Witteveen AB, et al. Correlates of prenatal and postnatal mother-to-infant bonding quality: a systematic review. PLoS One 2019; 14(9):e0222998.

66. Siqueira Barcelos R, da Silva dos Santos I, Matijasevich A, et al. Maternal depression is associated with injuries in children aged 2–4 years: the Pelotas 2004 Birth Cohort. Inj Prev 2019;25(3):222–7.

67. Abdollahi F, Abhari FR, Zarghami M. Post-partum depression effect on child health and development. Acta Med Iran 2017;55:109–14.

68. Myers S, Johns SE. Postnatal depression is associated with detrimental life-long and multi-generational impacts on relationship quality. PeerJ 2018;6:e4305.

69. Gutierrez-Galve L, Stein A, Hanington L, et al. Association of maternal and paternal depression in the postnatal period with offspring depression at age 18 years. JAMA Psychiatry 2019;76(3):290.

70. Ip P, Li TMH, Chan KL, et al. Associations of paternal postpartum depressive symptoms and infant development in a Chinese longitudinal study. Infant Behav Dev 2018;53:81–9.
71. Takehara K, Suto M, Kakee N, et al. Prenatal and early postnatal depression and child maltreatment among Japanese fathers. Child Abuse Negl 2017;70:231–9.
72. Stewart DE, Vigod SN. Postpartum depression: pathophysiology, treatment, and emerging therapeutics. Annu Rev Med 2019;70:183–96.
73. Kempler L, Sharpe L, Miller CB, et al. Do psychosocial sleep interventions improve infant sleep or maternal mood in the postnatal period? A systematic review and meta-analysis of randomised controlled trials. Sleep Med Rev 2016;29: 15–22.
74. McCurdy AP, Boulé NG, Sivak A, et al. Effects of exercise on mild-to-moderate depressive symptoms in the postpartum period: a meta-analysis. Obstet Gynecol 2017;129(6):1087–97.
75. Kołomańska-Bogucka D, Mazur-Bialy AI. Physical activity and the occurrence of postnatal depression—a systematic review. Medicina 2019;55(9):560–76.
76. Leger J, Letourneau N. New mothers and postpartum depression: a narrative review of peer support intervention studies. Health Soc Care Community 2015; 23(4):337–48.
77. O'Connor E, Senger CA, Henniger ML, et al. Interventions to prevent perinatal depression: evidence report and systematic review for the US Preventative Services Taskforce. JAMA 2019;321(6):588–601.
78. Stephens S, Ford E, Paudyal P, et al. Effectiveness of psychological interventions for postnatal depression in primary care: a meta-analysis. Ann Fam Med 2016; 14(5):463–72.
79. Frieder F, Fersh M, Hainline R, et al. Pharmacotherapy of postpartum depression: current approaches and novel drug development. CNS Drugs 2019;33:265–82.
80. De Crescenzo F, Perelli F, Armando M, et al. Selective serotonin reuptake inhibitors (SSRIs) for post-partum depression (PPD): a systematic review of randomized clinical trials. J Affect Disord 2014;152-154:39–44.
81. Molyneaux E, Howard LM, McGeown HR, et al. Antidepressant treatment for postnatal depression. Cochrane Database Syst Rev 2014;(9). https://doi.org/10.1002/14651858.CD002018.pub2.
82. US Food & Drug Administration. FDA approves first treatment for post-partum depression. FDA; 2019. Available at: https://www.fda.gov/news-events/press-announcements/fda-approves-first-treatment-post-partum-depression. Accessed November 29, 2020.
83. Sage Therapeutics. ZULRESSO™ (brexanolone) CIV Healthcare Professional Site. Zulresso. 2019. Available at: https://www.zulressohcp.com. Accessed November 29, 2020.
84. Meltzer-Brody S, Colquhoun H, Riesenberg R, et al. Brexanolone injection in postpartum depression: two multicentre, double-blind, randomised, placebo-controlled, phase 3 trials. Lancet 2018;392(10152):1058–70.
85. United States Securities and Exchange Commission. Form K-8 for Sage Therapeutics, Inc. US Securities Exchange Commission. 2019. Available at: https://www.sec.gov/Archives/edgar/data/1597553/000119312519079860/d721324d8k.htm. Accessed November 29, 2020.
86. Charandabi SM-A, Mirghafourvand M, Sanaati F. The effect of life style based education on the fathers' anxiety and depression during pregnancy and postpartum periods: a randomized controlled trial. Community Ment Health J 2017;53(4): 482–9.

87. Kroenke K, Spitzer RL, Williams JBW. The PHQ-9: validity of a brief depression severity measure. J Gen Intern Med 2001;16(9):606–13.
88. Rush AJ, First MB, Blacker D, editors. Handbook of psychiatric measures. 2nd edition. American Psychiatric Association; 2008.
89. Wang Y-P, Gorenstein C. Psychometric properties of the Beck Depression Inventory-II: a comprehensive review. Braz J Psychiatry 2013;35(4):416–31.
90. Simpson KR, Creehan PA, O'Brien-Abel N, et al. AWHONN perinatal nursing. 5th edition. Wolters Kluwer; 2021.

Early Recognition of Preventable Factors Associated with Delirium Saves Lives and Costs

Benjamin Smallheer, PhD, RN, ACNP-BC, FNP-BC, CCRN, CNE

KEYWORDS

- Delirium • Hyperactive • Hypoactive • Antipsychotics • Mortality

KEY POINTS

- Delirium can be characterized into 3 phenotypes: hyperactive, hypoactive, and mixed delirium.
- Delirium is characterized by 4 distinct features: (1) acute change or fluctuating course of mental status during the past 24 hours, (2) inattention, (3) an altered level of consciousness, and (4) disorganized thinking.
- An easy to administer bedside scoring tool is essential for the timely diagnosis of delirium.
- The goal for treating delirium is to manage behavioral disturbances while simultaneously finding and treating any causative medical disorders.

INTRODUCTION

Delirium is defined as an acute change or fluctuation in mental status with inattention accompanied either by disorganized thinking or an altered level of consciousness.[1] Its name is derived from the Latin word "delirare," which means "to go out of the furrow" or "crazy or deranged."[2] Although delirium is a common and serious problem in hospitalized older patients, its occurrence has been noted within the general community[3,4] and is associated with advancing age and the presence of dementia, infection, and prescribed medications.[4] The essential characteristics of delirium include impaired cognition and awareness representing a change from baseline attention and fluctuating in severity during the course of a day.[1,2] Individuals who develop delirium are at an increased risk for developing dementia, and thus may be more likely to require long-term care as they age. Because the number of individuals greater than 65 years of age has continued to increase, the natural result of longevity in this aging population has been the need for prolonged health services related to delirium.[3]

Duke University School of Nursing, 307 Trent Drive, DUMC Box 3322, Durham, NC 27710, USA
E-mail address: benjamin.smallheer@duke.edu

Nurs Clin N Am 56 (2021) 345–356
https://doi.org/10.1016/j.cnur.2021.04.002
0029-6465/21/© 2021 Elsevier Inc. All rights reserved.

nursing.theclinics.com

Delirium is associated with numerous costly and negative health care outcomes. Studies show that individuals who develop delirium have increased mortality, morbidity, psychological and physiologic distress, and prolonged hospital stays, and that the provision of their care has a negative effect on their personal and professional care givers.[3,5,6] The overall mortality rate for patients with delirium is 3 times higher than that of patients admitted with myocardial infarction or sepsis.[7] Leslie and Inouye[8] found that patients who experienced delirium had a 62% increased risk of mortality within 1 year after discharge, living an average of 274 days compared with 321 days among patients without delirium, a difference of 13% of a year.

EPIDEMIOLOGY AND INCIDENCE

The main characteristics of delirium are an acute loss of attention from baseline across a short period of time with fluctuation of symptoms throughout the day.[3] This presentation differs from that of dementia, which involves a disproportionate memory involvement that develops over time and a fairly preserved attention span.[3] Delirium can occur in any age; however, it has an increased prevalence and incidence in the elderly owing to impaired homeostasis, comorbid illnesses, dementia, and polypharmacy.[4] Classic symptoms of delirium resemble those of several other neuropsychiatric diseases, including dementia, psychosis, and depression.[3] These similarities often result in either a delayed diagnosis or misdiagnosis and poor management.[3]

Delirium is a relatively common disorder, affecting approximately 15% of older patients admitted to the hospital for medical care. In several general population studies, the prevalence of delirium was 1% to 2% in patients greater than 65 years old and ranged from 10% to 30% in hospitalized patients greater than 85 years old.[2,6,9] The incidence of delirium in patients who present to the emergency department for evaluation has been reported at 10% to 13% and increases to 22% to 42% in the inpatient setting.[7]

The causes of delirium are numerous and not completely understood. **Box 1** presents common causes and precipitating factors. The use of many medications including benzodiazepines and narcotic analgesics have been associated with increased incidence of delirium in aging patients.[3,9,10] One of the most widely used consensus criteria for medication use in older adults is known as the Beers criteria.[11,12] Based on expert consensus through an extensive literature review of geriatric care, clinical pharmacology, and psychopharmacology, the Beers criteria contain (a) an extensive list of medications known or believed to have an association with the incidence of delirium in older adults, (b) the rationale for inclusion in the criteria, (c) an official recommendation, (d) the quality of the evidence, and (e) the strength of the recommendation. The American Geriatrics Society[13] published an updated criteria in 2019. **Box 2** includes a list of common drug categories found within the criteria.

Other predisposing risk factors for delirium[3,4,9,14,15] include

- Advancing age
- Presence and severity of dementia
- Underlying cognitive impairment
- History of delirium
- Male sex
- Polypharmacy
- Depression
- Functional dependence
- Immobility
- Alcohol or illicit drug toxicity, overdose, or withdrawal
- Lack of sleep

Box 1
Common causes and precipitating factors for delirium[3,4,7,9,14–16]

Infection
- Urinary tract infection
- Sepsis
- Pneumonia

Metabolic and endocrine disturbances
- Electrolyte imbalance
- Dehydration
- Hypoglycemia and hyperglycemia

Changes in environment
- Visual impairment
- Auditory impairment

Underlying medical conditions
- Cardiovascular disease
- Hepatic disease
- Chronic renal failure

Neurologic
- Stroke or hemorrhage
- Seizures
- Meningitis and encephalitis

Trauma
- Head injury
- Heat stroke
- Burns
- Pain

Pulmonary
- Hypoxia
- Pulmonary failure
- Carbon monoxide poisoning

IMPACT OF DELIRIUM

The full effect of delirium beyond its financial impact remains unknown. A meta-analysis by Zhang and colleagues[17] found evidence that patients who experience delirium have longer length of stay in the intensive care unit (ICU) and require 7.22 days longer duration of mechanical ventilation during their ICU stay than nondelirious patients. Additionally, this prolonged need for mechanical ventilation and time in the ICU resulted in a longer overall in-hospital length of stay. The costs associated with prolonged mechanical ventilation in the United States range from $4 to $16 million per year, and the national financial burden of delirium on the United States health care system ranges from $38 billion to $152 billion each year.[2,7,8]

Delirium can affect every aspect of a patient's life. The effects of reliance on post-acute care and professional caregivers in addition to loss of independence and employment may never be measurable. In as many as 10% of all cases, the full cost of delirium on an individual, their family, or the health care system be may more than double what is known[18] because costs thought to be incidental or tangential to the primary diagnosis and treatment of the patient may not be captured readily. Delirium has been shown to lead to an acute decline in a patient's functional status.[19] Impairment may last up to 12 months and, for older patients, physical recovery has been found to be slower and less likely to return to baseline.[20] Although a shorter

---

Box 2
Common inappropriate medication categories for use in older adults[13]

Anticholinergics
- First-generation antihistamines
- Antiparkinsonian agents
- Antispasmodics

Antithrombotics

Anti-infectives

Cardiovascular agents
- Alpha$_1$ blockers
- Alpha$_2$ blockers, central
- Antiarrhythmic drugs

Central nervous system
- Antidepressants
- Antipsychotics
- Barbiturates
- Benzodiazepines
- Nonbenzodiazepine hypnotics

Endocrine
- Androgens
- Estrogens
- Growth hormone
- Insulin
- Sulfonylurea

Gastrointestinal agents
- Proton pump inhibitors

Pain medications
- Non–cyclo-oxygenase selective nonsteroidal anti-inflammatory drugs
- Skeletal muscle relaxants

---

duration of delirium is associated with better functional recovery, the severity of delirium does not seem to affect functional status independently.[19]

TYPES OF DELIRIUM

Delirium involves a range of cognitive changes and neuropsychiatric symptoms (eg, disturbances in motor behavior, sleep–wake cycle, affective expression, perception, and cognitive thinking), with the prominent features including inattention, disturbance of consciousness within short periods, and sudden change in psychotic features from baseline.[2,3] Cognitive changes such as memory loss, confusion, language disturbance, or emotional disturbance may not be easily detected in some patients such as those in the ICU,[2] in part owing to the use of high dose sedatives, opiates, or invasive therapies that impair the ability to communicate.

Delirium is a heterogeneous syndrome and has multiple phenotypes. Depending on the nature of the psychomotor disturbance and *Diagnostic and Statistical Manual of Mental Disorders* (DSM), fifth edition specifier definition, delirium is frequently classified as

1. Hyperactive (characterized by increased psychomotor activity that may be accompanied by mood lability, agitation, and/or refusal to cooperate with medical care);
2. Hypoactive (characterized by decreased psychomotor activity that may be accompanied by sluggishness, lethargy, or stupor); or

3. Mixed (characterized by normal psychomotor activity with disturbed attention and awareness, or rapid fluctuation between hyperactive and hypoactive states of delirium).[1,7]

Hyperactive delirium is characterized by motor agitation, restlessness, and sometimes aggressiveness.[7,20] Symptoms of hyperactive delirium[15] include

- Acting disoriented
- Anxiety
- Hallucinations
- Rambling
- Rapid changes in emotion
- Restlessness
- Trouble concentrating

Hypoactive delirium is characterized by

- Motor retardation
- Apathy
- Slowing of speech, and
- The appearance of being sedated.20

The most common subtype, hypoactive delirium can be missed easily owing to its subtle clinical presentation; it carries the worst prognosis and has been associated with poorer in-hospital and long-term mortality.[7] It is predicted that up to 75% of people with delirium experience hypoactive delirium.[15] Symptoms of hypoactive delirium[15] include

- Apathy
- Decreased responsiveness
- Flat affect
- Laziness
- Withdrawal

Mixed delirium is a combination of hyperactive and hypoactive delirum.[7,20] Patients often display few or no motor symptoms but experience significant cognitive symptoms, and may switch between hyper- and hypoactive symptoms over time.

COMMON SCORING TOOLS

Recognizing delirium symptoms to obtain an accurate diagnosis can be challenging. Nurses have identified 3 major barriers to assessment for delirium: (1) the difficulty of evaluating delirium in intubated patients, (2) the inability to complete delirium assessment of sedated patients, and (3) the complexity of many delirium assessment tools. The early detection of delirium is particularly challenging because delirium presents as a multifactorial disorder with varied clinical manifestations that differ based on patient population and hospital setting.[21] It is estimated that delirium remains undiagnosed in 75% of patients in the absence of structured detection tools.[2] In situations where early detection and diagnosis are hindered, patients experience further decline, resulting in persistent functional and cognitive loss.

Although many scales exist to detect and evaluate delirium, the DSM currently endorses 5 validated screening tools for adult patients[1]: the Confusion Assessment Method (CAM)-ICU,[22] the Intensive Care Delirium Screening Checklist,[23] the Delirium Detection Score (DDS),[24] the Nursing Delirium Screening Scale (Nu-DESC),[25] and the Neelon and Champagne Confusion Scale (NEECHAM).[26] Other validated delirium tools are listed in **Box 3**.

Box 3
Other delirium assessment instruments[7]

- Single Question in Delirium[5,6]
  - Is this patient more confused than before? Yes/No
- Brief CAM[27]
- Ultrabrief 2-item Bedside Test[10]
  - Please tell me the day of the week.
  - Please tell me the months of the year backward, say December as your first month. (If incorrect in either question, an additional screening is necessary.)
- Delirium Triage Screen[27]
  - Altered level of consciousness by the Richmond Agitation-Sedation Scale[a]
  - Can you spell the word "LUNCH" backwards? (If incorrect in either question, additional assessment is necessary.)
- 4AT[28]
  - Alertness normal (0)/abnormal (+4)
  - Age, date of birth, place, current year. No mistake (0)/one mistake (+1)/greater than 2 mistakes or untestable (+2)
  - Attention (month of the year backwards). Lists $\geq$7 months (0)/starts but <7 months or refuse (+1)/untestable (+2)
  - Acute change or fluctuating course. Yes (+4)/No (0)
    (Score 0 normal, score 1–3 possible cognitive impairment, $\geq$4 possible delirium and/or cognitive impairment)
- Brief CAM[27]
  - Feature 1[b]: Altered mental status or fluctuating course
  - Feature 2[b]: Can you name the months backwards from December to July?
  - Feature 3[c]: Altered level of consciousness (by the Richmond Agitation-Sedation Scale)
  - Feature 4[c]: Disorganized thinking
    1. Will a stone float on water?
    2. Are there fish in the sea?
    3. Does 1 pound weigh more than 2 pounds?
    4. Can you use a hammer to pound a nail?
       Command: "Hold up [this many] fingers," and "Now do the same thing with the other hand."

[a]The Richmond Agitation-Sedation Scale is a 10-point scale, with 4 levels of anxiety or agitation (+1 to +4 [combative]), 1 level to denote a calm and alert state (0), and 5 levels of sedation (−1 to −5) culminating in unarousable (−5). [b]Feature 1 and 2 need to be abnormal for delirium. [c]If feature 1 and 2 are abnormal, the presence of abnormal feature 3 or feature 4 meets criteria for delirium.

Reproduced from S. Lee et al./American Journal of Emergency Medicine 38 (2020) 349–357351.

Before a patient can be screened for delirium, a thorough assessment of their level of consciousness should be undertaken using an established scale such as the Richmond Agitation-Sedation Scale.[2] A subsequent diagnosis should be based on history taking, a discussion with caretakers and nursing teams, a and review of medical records, and can be supported further using diagnostic tools and scales, such as the CAM[29] or the 3-minute delirium assessment (3D-CAM).[30] The CAM defines delirium in terms of 4 diagnostic features: (1) acute change or fluctuating course of mental status during the past 24 hours, (2) inattention, (3) altered level of consciousness (currently measured as the Richmond Agitation and Sedation Scale level), and (4) disorganized thinking. A diagnosis of delirium requires the presence of features 1 and 2 in addition to 3 and/or 4. The tool requires 5 minutes to complete, is considered easy to administer, and can be used with patients who have hearing and visual disturbances.[22]

The CAM-ICU[22] is an adaptation of the CAM, which was originally developed to allow a nonpsychiatrist to assess delirium at the bedside, and is used to assess delirium in patients in the ICU. It consists of the same 4 features as the CAM; however, it takes into consideration the possibility that a critically ill patient may be unable to speak. Therefore, it allows for the use of assessment aids such as the Richmond Agitation-Sedation Scale or the Glasgow Coma Scale to be used to determine acute onset or fluctuating course (feature 1), and the attention screening examination to be used to evaluate for inattention (feature 2). In addition, specifically developed standardized questions evaluate for disorganized thinking (feature 3).[22]

The Intensive Care Delirium Screening Checklist[23] is a screening checklist of 8 items based on the 4 DSM features of delirium. It further delineates the 4 features to enable the evaluation of potentially unstable or intubated patients by incorporating examination findings of the following[31]:

Altered level of consciousness	Inattention	Disorientation
Hallucinations/delusions	Sleep/wake cycle disturbance	Symptom fluctuation
Inappropriate speech or mood	Psychomotor agitation/retardation	

The DDS[24] was developed to provide a monitoring system that can be used easily with both intubated and nonintubated patients in the ICU. This scale was created by modifying the Clinical Withdrawal Assessment for Alcohol, which is used to evaluate alcohol withdrawal syndrome. The DDS is composed of 8 criteria: agitation, anxiety, hallucination, orientation, seizures, tremors, paroxysmal sweating, and altered sleep–wake rhythm. These criteria are useful for diagnosing and assessing the degree of delirium and for guiding treatment.[32]

The Nu-DESC[25] is a 5-item scale that can be quickly completed by the bedside clinician through observation. There are other delirium scales that do not require patient participation and are adapted to the fluctuating nature of delirium; however, these are either not fully validated or not based on the DSM criteria for delirium.[1] The Nu-DESC includes the 4 DMS features of disorientation, inappropriate behavior, inappropriate communication, and illusions and hallucinations, and it adds the category of unusual psychomotor retardation to better account for the hypoactive form of delirium.

The NEECHAM[26] was developed to facilitate rapid and unobtrusive assessment and monitoring of acute confusion. Although at the time of its development the DSM-IV had recently been released, there was concern that instances of delirium were not being detected because not all patients were manifesting the criteria required for diagnosis; therefore, the NEECHAM was developed for bedside assessment to identify early changes or subclinical manifestations of disturbed information processing. On this scale, the patient's level of processing information, level of behavior, and physiologic condition over a 24-hour period inform a rating that classifies the patient as (a) nondelirious (normal), (b) at risk, (c) having early to mild confusion (mild confusion), or (d) having moderate to severe confusion.[33]

TREATMENT OF DELIRIUM

The early recognition of delirium can facilitate timely treatment. Hyperactive and hypoactive delirium are managed in different ways, so an accurate diagnosis is essential. Hyperactive delirium treatment often includes antipsychotic medications and the use of physical restraints owing to a patient's motor agitation and/or tendency to pull at lines and tubes, impeding care; in contrast, the use of antipsychotic medications in patients with the hypoactive subtype is generally avoided.[20] Mixed delirium often goes unrecognized until the patient displays and receives treatment for hyperactive symptoms. Overall, the goal of delirium treatment is to manage behavioral disturbances while simultaneously finding and treating any causative medical disorders.

Nonpharmacologic Interventions

Because delirium is a multifactorial syndrome, preventive strategies should be included within the patient's plan of care and ideally should focus on a multicomponent protocol. Using nonpharmacologic interventions whenever possible can minimize the risk of drug–drug interactions and adverse drug reactions. The use of nonpharmacological interventions may also decrease the risk of worsening delirium among elderly patients by up to 40%.[2] Further strategies that have been shown to significantly decrease delirium severity include efforts to decrease overall hospital stay; limit the frequency of room changes; facilitate family support; ensure the presence of clocks, unobstructed windows, and reading glasses if needed; and limit the use of medical or physical restraints.[2] Other first-line interventions that are low risk and consistent with standards for quality care include the following[7]:

- Reorientation
- Behavioral intervention
- Hydration
- Hearing and vision competency
- Clear instructions and frequent eye contact
- Verbal de-escalation

Interventions should be taken to minimize the level of noise within the patient's care area, such as discontinuing the use of unnecessary monitors or equipment, silencing or removing telephones, adjusting alarm volumes to the safest minimum level, and implementing earplugs at bedtime. These interventions have been shown to lead to better sleep and improved delirium prevention, especially if used within 48 hours of admission.[2] Finally, the care team can implement bundle interventions such as the ABCDE bundle,[34] which prompts the care team to regularly address the following: Awakening and Breathing, Coordination of daily sedation and ventilator removal trials, Choice of sedation and analgesic exposure, Delirium monitoring and management, and Early mobility and Exercise.[34]

Pharmacologic Interventions

The goal of pharmacologic therapy should be to control agitation and calm the patient while avoiding oversedation.[35] It is preferred that this goal be accomplished through oral administration of medication rather than by injection to minimize discomfort, agitation, and hemodynamic instability or arrhythmia caused by increased agitation and/or anxiety.[7] As a general guideline, benzodiazepines should be avoided except for selected indications such as alcohol withdrawal because this drug class has been associated with worsened confusion, significantly more delirium, and worse outcomes.[36,37] The clinician should also consider the appropriateness of pharmacologic therapies to the care environment of the patient. A Cochrane review concluded that the use of antipsychotics did not show strong evidence of treatment effects outside of the ICU as compared with their use on patients receiving critical care.[38]

Antipsychotic agents are generally used to treat severe agitation associated with delirium. The most frequently used antipsychotic medications for treating delirium include the first-generation antipsychotic medication haloperidol (75%–80%) and atypical antipsychotics (35%–40%).[2] The use of typical antipsychotics has been questioned owing to a high prevalence of extrapyramidal symptoms, and second-generation antipsychotics have a lower risk of these side effects when used for delirium.[2,7] Second-generation antipsychotics used in the management and treatment of delirium include olanzapine, risperidone, quetiapine, and ziprasidone.[2,7] Nurses should be aware of the potential for QT prolongation with many of these medications and should monitor the patient's electrocardiogram.

The use of alpha-2 agonist medications such as dexmedetomidine have proven effective in managing anxiety and pain and for decreasing the incidence of delirium in critically ill patients.[37] This drug class has a minimal effect on respiratory effort while helping to maintain a lower heart rate, resulting in minimal hemodynamic fluctuations, lower energy expenditure, and less global cerebral insult.[2]

The following stepwise approach to pharmacologic treatment should be considered[39]:

1. Provide nonpharmacologic/pharmacologic supportive measures including
   a. Reorientation and reassurance
   b. Hydration
   c. Mobilization
   d. Avoidance of restraints
   e. Reduction of stimulation
   f. Pain management
2. Review medications and evaluate for potential causes
3. Ask whether the patient's behavior is interfering with care or safety
   a. If yes, institute pharmacologic interventions
   b. If not, continue nonpharmacologic interventions

SUMMARY

Delirium is a complex condition that has a significant impact on patient outcomes and health care costs. The DSM-5 recognizes delirium as having 4 distinct features: (1) acute change or fluctuating course of mental status during the past 24 hours, (2) inattention, (3) altered level of consciousness, and (4) disorganized thinking. The difficulty of obtaining a timely diagnosis presents one of the greatest challenges to the treatment of delirium. Several tools have been developed to aid the early diagnosis of delirium, 5 of which are currently endorsed by the DSM: the CAM-ICU, the Intensive Care Delirium Screening Checklist, the DDS, the Nu-DESC, and the NEECHAM. After a diagnosis of delirium, a combination of nonpharmacologic and pharmacologic interventions should be simultaneously instituted to control agitation and calm the patient while causation is explored.

CLINICS CARE POINTS

- Individuals who develop delirium are at an increased risk of 1 year mortality as well as developing dementia.
- Classic symptoms of delirium resemble those of several other neuropsychiatric diseases, including dementia, psychosis, and depression.
- Delirium may present as hyperactive, hypoactive, or mixed delirium.
- Hypoactive is the most common subtype, and is easily missed owing to its subtle clinical presentation.
- Early recognition of delirium is essential to facilitate timely treatment.

- The goal of delirium treatment is to manage behavioral disturbances through the simultaneous use of nonpharmacologic and pharmacologic means, while concurrently finding and treating any causative medical disorders.

DISCLOSURE

The author has no disclosures regarding the support or work of this article. The author has no conflicts of interest on this topic or any of the works cited within.

REFERENCES

1. American Psychiatric Association. Diagnostic and statistical manual of mental disorders. 5th edition. American Psychiatric Association; 2013.
2. Arumugam S, El-Menyar A, Al-Hassani A, et al. Delirium in the intensive care unit. J Emerg Trauma Shock 2017;10(1):37.
3. Ritter SRF, Cardoso AF, Lins MMP, et al. Underdiagnosis of delirium in the elderly in acute care hospital settings: lessons not learned: delirium diagnosis: lessons not learned. Psychogeriatrics 2018;18(4):268–75.
4. Raju K, Coombe-Jones M. An overview of delirium for the community and hospital clinician: delirium. Prog Neurol Psychiatry 2015;19(6):23–7.
5. McCleary E, Cumming P. Improving early recognition of delirium using SQiD (Single Question to identify Delirium): a hospital based quality improvement project. BMJ Qual Improv Rep 2015;4(1). u206598.w2653.
6. Sands M, Dantoc B, Hartshorn A, et al. Single question in delirium (SQiD): testing its efficacy against psychiatrist interview, the Confusion Assessment Method and the memorial delirium assessment scale. Palliat Med 2010;24(6):561–5.
7. Lee S, Gottlieb M, Mulhausen P, et al. Recognition, prevention, and treatment of delirium in emergency department: an evidence-based narrative review. Am J Emerg Med 2020;38(2):349–57.
8. Leslie DL, Inouye SK. The importance of delirium: economic and societal costs. J Am Geriatr Soc 2011;59:S241–3.
9. Kim H, Chung S, Joo Y, et al. The major risk factors for delirium in a clinical setting. Neuropsychiatr Dis Treat 2016;12:1787–93.
10. Fick DM, Inouye SK, Guess J, et al. Preliminary development of an ultrabrief two-item bedside test for delirium: two-item bedside test for delirium. J Hosp Med 2015;10(10):645–50.
11. Beers MH. Explicit criteria for determining potentially inappropriate medication use by the elderly: an update. Arch Intern Med 1997;157(14):1531.
12. Beers MH. Explicit criteria for determining inappropriate medication use in nursing home residents. Arch Intern Med 1991;151(9):1825.
13. The 2019 American Geriatrics Society Beers Criteria® Update Expert Panel. American Geriatrics Society 2019 updated AGS Beers Criteria® for potentially inappropriate medication use in older adults. J Am Geriatr Soc 2019;67(4):674–94.
14. Kumar PJ, Clark M, Feather A, editors. Kumar and Clark's clinical medicine. 9th edition. Elsevier; 2017.
15. Delirium. Cleveland clinic website. 2020. Available at: https://my.clevelandclinic.org/health/diseases/15252-delirium. Accessed December 23, 2020.
16. Kanich W, Brady WJ, Huff JS, et al. Altered mental status: evaluation and etiology in the ED. Am J Emerg Med 2002;20(7):613–7.
17. Zhang Z, Pan L, Ni H. Impact of delirium on clinical outcome in critically ill patients: a meta-analysis. Gen Hosp Psychiatry 2013;35(2):105–11.

18. Caplan GA, Teodorczuk A, Streatfeild J, et al. The financial and social costs of delirium. Eur Geriatr Med 2020;11(1):105–12.
19. Boettger S, Breitbart W, Jenewein J, et al. Delirium and functionality: the impact of delirium on the level of functioning. Eur J Psychiatry 2014;28(2):86–95.
20. van Velthuijsen EL, Zwakhalen SMG, Mulder WJ, et al. Detection and management of hyperactive and hypoactive delirium in older patients during hospitalization: a retrospective cohort study evaluating daily practice. Int J Geriatr Psychiatry 2018;33(11):1521–9.
21. Johnson K, Diana S, Todd J, et al. Early recognition of delirium in trauma patients. Intensive Crit Care Nurs 2016;34:28–32.
22. Ely EW, Inouye SK, Bernard GR, et al. Delirium in mechanically ventilated patients: validity and reliability of the Confusion Assessment Method for the intensive care unit (CAM-ICU). JAMA 2001;286(21):2703.
23. Bergeron N, Dubois M-J, Dumont M, et al. Intensive care delirium screening checklist: evaluation of a new screening tool. Intensive Care Med 2001;27(5): 859–64.
24. Otter H, Martin J, Bäsell K, et al. Validity and reliability of the DDS for severity of delirium in the ICU. Neurocrit Care 2005;2(2):150–8.
25. Gaudreau J-D, Gagnon P, Harel F, et al. Fast, systematic, and continuous delirium assessment in hospitalized patients: the Nursing Delirium Screening Scale. J Pain Symptom Manage 2005;29(4):368–75.
26. Neelon VJ, Champagne MT, Carlson JR, et al. The NEECHAM Confusion Scale: construction, validation, and clinical testing. Nurs Res 1996;45(6):324–30. Available at: https://journals.lww.com/nursingresearchonline/Fulltext/1996/11000/The_NEECHAM_Confusion_Scale__Construction,.2.aspx.
27. Han JH, Wilson A, Vasilevskis EE, et al. Diagnosing delirium in older emergency department patients: validity and reliability of the delirium triage screen and the brief Confusion Assessment Method. Ann Emerg Med 2013;62(5):457–65.
28. Bellelli G, Morandi A, Davis DHJ, et al. Corrigendum to 'Validation of the 4AT, a new instrument for rapid delirium screening: a study in 234 hospitalised older people. Age Ageing 2015;44(1):175.
29. Inouye SK. Clarifying confusion: the Confusion Assessment Method. A new method for detection of delirium. Ann Intern Med 1990;113(12):941.
30. Marcantonio ER, Ngo LH, O'Connor M, et al. 3D-CAM: derivation and validation of a 3-minute diagnostic interview for CAM-defined delirium: a cross-sectional diagnostic test study. Ann Intern Med 2014;161(8):554.
31. Devlin JW, Marquis F, Riker RR, et al. Combined didactic and scenario-based education improves the ability of intensive care unit staff to recognize delirium at the bedside. Crit Care 2008;12(1):R19.
32. Carvalho JPLM, de Almeida ARP, Gusmao-Flores D. Delirium rating scales in critically ill patients: a systematic literature review. Rev Bras Ter Intensiva 2013;25(2): 148–54.
33. Van Rompaey B, Schuurmans MJ, Shortridge-Baggett LM, et al. A comparison of the CAM-ICU and the NEECHAM Confusion Scale in intensive care delirium assessment: an observational study in non-intubated patients. Crit Care 2008; 12(1):R16.
34. Morandi A, Brummel NE, Ely EW. Sedation, delirium and mechanical ventilation: the 'ABCDE' approach. Curr Opin Crit Care 2011;17(1):43–9.
35. Zun L, Wilson MP, Nordstrom K. Treatment goal for agitation: sedation or calming. Ann Emerg Med 2017;70(5):751–2.

36. Lonergan E, Luxenberg J, Areosa Sastre A. Benzodiazepines for delirium. [Intervention review]. Cochrane Dementia and Cognitive Improvement Group. Cochrane Database Syst Rev 2009;2009(4):CD006379.
37. Pandharipande PP, Pun BT, Herr DL, et al. Effect of sedation with Dexmedetomidine vs Lorazepam on acute brain dysfunction in mechanically ventilated patients: the MENDS randomized controlled trial. JAMA 2007;298(22):2644.
38. Burry L, Mehta S, Perreault MM, et al. Antipsychotics for treatment of delirium in hospitalised non-ICU patients. Cochrane Dementia and Cognitive Improvement Group. Cochrane Database Syst Rev 2018;6(6):CD005594.
39. Francis J. Delirium and acute confusional states: prevention, treatment, and prognosis. In: Wilterdink J, ed. UpToDate. UpToDate Inc. Available at: https://www.uptodate.com/contents/delirium-and-acute-confusional-states-prevention-treatment-and-prognosis. Accessed December 30, 2020.

Advocating for Multimodal Pain Management and Reducing the Need for Opioids in the Acute and Chronic Pain Setting

Janelle M. Delle, DNP, MSN, ACNP-BC[a], Cheryl Gazley, FNP-BC[b],*

KEYWORDS

- Acute pain • Chronic pain • Opioid misuse • Multimodal therapy
- Health care advocate

KEY POINTS

- Multimodal pain management is becoming more of an effective and safe way to treat postoperative pain in the acute care setting versus using opioids alone.
- The opioid epidemic has led to a rise in opioid prescriptions and patient consumption, which accounted for an increase in opioid misuse and accidental overdoses.
- The use of combination therapies assists in targeting different pain receptors to help achieve adequate pain management, thus using less opioids.
- Health care providers must serve as patient advocates, performing adequate physical assessments and interventions to ensure the patient receives optimum patient care through the use of appropriate analgesics, and through a multimodal approach in postoperative care.
- Multimodal approaches have been shown to reduce hospital stay, health care costs, and overuse of resources, and increase patient satisfaction.
- Focusing on a multimodal pain approach assists in lowering the prevalence of opioid-induced misuse and deaths and sets about putting an end to the opioid epidemic.

INTRODUCTION

Many Americans suffer from acute and chronic pain, whether from an illness, traumatic injury, recent surgery, arthritis, or even cancer pain. Pain stimulates the nervous

a Vanderbilt University Medical Center, 1211 Medical Center Drive, D-2106 MCN, Nashville, TN 37232, USA; b Interventional Pain Center, 353 New Shackle Island Road, Suite 101-A, Hendersonville, TN 37075, USA
* Corresponding author.
E-mail address: Janelle.delle@vumc.org

Nurs Clin N Am 56 (2021) 357–367
https://doi.org/10.1016/j.cnur.2021.04.003
0029-6465/21/© 2021 Elsevier Inc. All rights reserved.

system sending signals to your brain that something unpleasant is occurring in your body. Pain can be constant, intermittent, sharp, dull, stabbing, throbbing, burning, and so forth, all pointing to an uncomfortable feeling and disrupting homeostasis. Pain can affect one's physical, emotional, and environmental factors, especially in chronic pain, which exists longer than 3 months. Chronic pain is difficult to treat because some patients become unaffected by certain pain medications, thus prompting the prescriber to either increase medication doses or add additional medications, thus leading to polypharmacy.[1] When treating chronic pain, providers must make a distinction between cancer pain and noncancer pain, and which treatment path to take for effective and safe pain management.[2] The annual cost of medical expenses and lost wages related to pain is excessively higher than treatment of diabetes, heart disease, or cancer-related medical costs.[3] In a 2011 report by the Institute of Medicine cost estimates of chronic pain were around $560 billion, in which $100 billion was spent treating spinal pain, including surgery.

Given the concern for opioid abuse and overdose, many pain prescribers are adopting a multimodal approach to pain management.[4] Multimodal pain management is becoming more of an effective and safe way to treat postoperative pain in the acute care setting versus using opioids alone. They further state that roughly 116 people die every day from opioid overuse in the Unites States. Opioid usage may start in the acute care setting and continue months into the postoperative phase, leading to opioid abuse. Nurses are at the forefront of this issue because they are the ones to administer pain medications in the acute care setting.[5] Nursing, which goes back several centuries, has been an actively involved profession where a person provides care for the sick patient to restore homeostasis in a safe and responsible environment. One of the most common responsibilities of a trained nurse is acting as patient advocate, taking charge of keeping their patient's safe and out of harm's way, practicing ethically and judiciously acting in the patient's best interest. With the recent opioid epidemic in the United States within the last few years, nurses must ensure that post-surgical patients are not receiving an excess number of opioids that could potentially lead to an accidental drug overdose or death, not excluding those patients who end up relying on opioids for an extended period of time for adequate pain control. Health care providers are responsible for performing adequate physical assessments and interventions to ensure the patient receives optimum patient care including the safe and effective use of analgesics in postoperative care.[6] According to the Centers for Disease Control and Prevention,[7] since 1999, more than 75,000 people have died of a drug overdose, with 47,000 deaths in 2018, in which 32% of these deaths were from prescribed opioids. The rate of opioid prescriptions in the United States heightened and then leveled off from 2010 to 2012, and continues to decline; however, the number of opioids contained in morphine milligram equivalents per prescription is three times higher than it was in 1999. Morphine milligram equivalents refers to an opioid's equivalency to morphine and is often used to assess the likelihood of potential overdose in the amount of the prescribed opioid that the patient takes for a given time. Another term used is morphine equivalent daily dose (MEDD), which is the formula used to provide the number of morphine equivalents a patient is taking per day or month. This is done by comparing pain medication the patient is taking with the strength of morphine and giving it a number. According to research, 22 states in the United States have at least one kind of MEDD policy.[8] The most common type of MEDD policy is state guidelines, which currently includes 14 states. Other types include prior authorizations, which currently includes four states. Other policies include legislative acts (three states), claim denials (two states), and alert systems (currently in two states). Most of the policies omit certain groups of opioid users, typically acute pain patients, burn patients, sickle cell patients, cancer-related pain, and patients who are terminally ill. MEDD numbers can vary from state to state, although frequently range from 30 to 300 mg. The higher MEDD thresholds largely correspond to a more restrictive policy, such as claim denial, whereas the lower thresholds usually correspond to a less restrictive policy, such as a guideline. MEDD policies have become more prevalent in recent years, although the threshold levels can vary greatly, and policy structure can lead to a deficiency of consensus. This information shows that more states should put more emphasis on such policies to crack down on overprescribing of opioids.

The rise in opioid prescriptions and patient consumption led to an increase in opioid misuse and accidental overdoses, with the highest incidence occurring in 2014. In 2015, overdose deaths rose to 33,000 in the United States, also leading to an increased amount of deaths from heroin (increased to 20%) and fentanyl (increased to 72%) between 2014 and 2015, likely related to easy accessibility and low cost. Most of the population who abuse opioids do not have a medical prescription.[9] Patients who misuse opioids may be at increased risk of developing psychological effects, such as depression, anxiety, bipolar disorder, and even alcohol abuse problems, all of which is associated with increased health care services and costs.[10]

Prescription opioids are often given for acute and chronic pain; however, these can carry serious risks and unpleasant side effects including constipation, nausea, vomiting, oversedation, overdose (intentional or accidental), addiction, and potentially death. It is important to ascertain the need for opioids, especially in the acute care setting. Consumption of opioids for an extended period of time should warrant provider discussions to consider alternative medications, such as multimodal therapy. It is important for health care providers to understand what has been practiced in the past with the use of opioid therapy to improve what is implemented for success in the future with a multimodal pain approach. Furthermore, it is essential to understand how to treat pain from the lens of acute versus chronic, versus those patients who suffer with pain from cancer-related causes.[2]

Multimodal pain management has become widely used in the acute care setting because it is a combination of multiple pharmacologic medications from different drug classes, used together to help reduce the amount of pain in a given time, especially in the acute care setting. The goal of multimodal pain management is to achieve adequate pain management without using an increased number of opioids, hence, using a combination of medications with different modes of action to achieve adequate pain control and less side effects.[11] Combination drug classes may include nonsteroidal anti-inflammatory drugs (NSAIDs), acetaminophen, opioids, α_2-agonists, N-methyl-D-aspartate (NMDA) receptor antagonists, anticonvulsants, or local anesthetic blocks.[12] Multimodal approaches have been shown to reduce length of hospital stay, costs, overuse of resources, and an increase in patient satisfaction. Furthermore, advocation for nonpharmacologic therapies, such as cupping, acupuncture, acupressure, or deep-tissue massage, has been investigated. Using a multimodal drug therapy approach coupled with nonpharmacologic therapies can greatly reduce the need for opioid-induced pain control.[13]

HISTORY

Although the United States has seen a rise in the use and misuse of opioids in the last two decades, the opioid epidemic dates back to ancient civilization with the consumption of plants for medicinal purposes. The oil and seed extracts of the poppy plant, known as "joy plant," was one of the first "opioids" used for pain management. Moving forward to the 1800s, heroin was readily available to purchase over-the-counter and in massive quantity. By the early 1970s there were around 200,000 heroin addicts in the United States, which prompted the US government to establish the Controlled Substance Act to regulate the manufacture, use, and distribution of certain drugs.[3] This federal US drug policy began placing medications into five categories (Schedule I-V) to determine risk of abuse, with the highest potential for abuse to lowest. All medications considered "controlled substances" by the Food and Drug Administration are organized into five categories to determine medical purpose for use and dependency potential. Schedule I controlled substances, such as heroin, have no medical purpose and have a high risk of abuse. On the other end of the spectrum, Schedule V includes those over-the-counter medications with the lowest potential for abuse or dependence, such as antitussives (eg, Robitussin AC) (**Box 1**).[14] The act of organizing certain drugs into scheduled categories helps guide health care providers to safely prescribe necessary medications that treat acute and chronic pain; however, there are still instances of overprescribing and potential for abuse with opioid painkillers.[15]

Many health care providers that treat those patients who suffer from chronic pain have long prescribed opioids before referring to pain clinics for further interventional approaches.[13] It is important for providers to ascertain patient expectations when initiating opioid prescribed therapy for chronic pain and those surgical patients who may start off with a multimodal pain approach in the perioperative setting. From 2017 to 2018, the opioid epidemic began to take a positive turn. Initiation of prescription drug monitoring programs, such as the Drug Enforcement Administration, began to enforce strict laws and regulations of controlled substances to cut down on opioid misuse and overdose. Additionally, educational programs became more readily

---

Box 1
Schedule of controlled substances, examples

Schedule I (no current accepted medical use)
- Heroin
- Cannabis
- Lysergic acid diethylamide (LSD)

Schedule II (high potential for abuse)
- Hydromorphone
- Methadone
- Oxycodone
- Fentanyl

Schedule III (potential for abuse)
- Tylenol with codeine
- Suboxone
- Ketamine
- Phendimetrazine

Schedule IV (low potential for abuse)
- Xanax
- Soma
- Klonopin
- Lorazepam

Schedule V (low potential for abuse)
- Robitussin AC
- Ezogabine

available with changes in state regulations and suppression of opioid production, which marked the beginning of change for the opioid epidemic in the United States. With this significant movement, federal expenses for recovery programs increased from \$599 million to \$2.1 billion.[3] Furthermore, an additional resource to help crack down on the opioid epidemic is through the organization of the National Safety Council. The National Safety Council is a nonprofit mission-based organization that provides safe practice toolkits to companies to ensure that employees are using the resources provided to them to live safer, fuller lives, thus increasing workplace productivity. This safety toolkit offers a wide variety of resources to include assisting in decreasing opioid abuse and overdose by mandating safe practice education to those providers prescribing opioids while implementing prescribing guidelines, integrating prescription drug monitoring programs into inpatient and outpatient settings with tracking and sharing capabilities through online resources, such as the Drug Enforcement Administration, and most importantly providing those resources for opioid abuse treatment programs.[16]

DEFINITIONS

Pain refers to an unpleasant feeling that stems from the nervous system that causes a person to feel symptoms, such as sharp, dull, throbbing, burning, tingling, or stabbing. It may be localized to a specific part of the body or generalized to a specific area. Most of the time it is easy to diagnose, but not in all cases. Pain alone may be influenced by psychological, biologic, or social factors.[1] Acute pain is defined as pain of recent onset and probable limited duration. It usually has an identifiable temporal and causal relationship to injury or disease.[17] Chronic pain differs from acute pain because it may last for weeks, months, or even years. It may be caused by an initial injury from trauma, any type of sprain, cancer, arthritis, or certain autoimmune disorders.[18]

Multimodal pain management refers to using pharmacologic and nonpharmacologic methods to treat acute and chronic pain. Nonopioid pharmacologic methods include using a combination of medications from different drug classes, with a goal of targeting various pain receptors to achieve adequate pain relief, thus using less opioids. The most commonly used multimodal medications include analgesics (eg, acetaminophen), NSAIDs, local anesthetics (eg, limb blocks and α_2-agonists), NMDA antagonists, and anticonvulsants (**Box 2**).[4] Nonpharmacologic methods include guided imagery, deep-tissue massage, acupuncture, acupressure, trigger point injections, hypnosis, heat/cold therapy, music therapy, and meditation.[19]

The opioid epidemic refers to a period in time around 2017 when the Department of Health and Human Services saw a surge in the amount of prescription opioids that were prescribed, which led to addiction, abuse, misuse, and even deaths from this class of pain medications. A public health emergency was soon declared with a plan laid out to combat the opioid crisis.[20]

BACKGROUND

Given stricter state laws and regulations with the production of and prescribing of opioids, there still remains a gap in standardizing opioid prescribing practices. According to the Centers for Disease Control and Prevention, roughly 20% of patients with non-cancer pain or acute and chronic pain who present to their primary medical provider receive a prescription for an opioid. More than 250 million opioid prescriptions were written in 2012, which is equivalent for every person in the United States to have a single filled pill bottle. Furthermore, per capita, opioid prescriptions rose to 7.3% from the year 2007 to 2012. The initiation of multimodal pain therapy has played a huge role in

---

Box 2
Multimodal drugs commonly used

Analgesics
- Acetaminophen (APAP)
- NSAIDs, aspirin (salicylates)
- Opioids (oxycodone, morphine)

NSAIDS
- Ibuprofen
- Naproxen
- Diclofenac
- Celecoxib

Limb blocks
- Epidural anesthesia: bupivacaine, lidocaine, chloroprocaine
- Peripheral nerve block: bupivacaine, lidocaine, ropivacaine

α_2-Agonists
- Guanfacine
- Clonidine
- Tizanidine

NMDA receptor antagonists
- Amantadine
- Memantine
- Ketamine

Anticonvulsants
- Gabapentin
- Pregabalin

---

reducing overprescribing of opioids and shifted toward a downward slope on the continuum within the opioid pandemic.[21] Multimodal pain therapy allows medications from different drug classes to work on different pain receptors to help achieve safe and adequate pain control, while also decreasing opioid-related side effects.

Researchers discuss a retrospective study[22] by the Michigan Opioid Prescribing Engagement Network in coordination with the Michigan Surgical Quality Collaborative in an independent community hospital in Michigan before and after initiation of hospital-wide educational programs and state legislation changes on safer opioid prescribing practices. Inclusion criteria included opioid-naive adult postoperative patients who underwent one of the five most common minimally invasive surgical procedures including an appendectomy, cholecystectomy, inguinal hernia repair, and breast lumpectomy with or without sentinel lymph node biopsy from 2015 to 2017. Exclusion criteria included pregnant patients, any of the minimally invasive procedures that turned into open procedures, any patients using prescribed opioids in the last 90 days, any history of opioid misuse or abuse, and any missing postoperative prescription information within the medical record. The hospital-wide educational program used the Michigan Opioid Prescribing Engagement Network recommended dose, which was 75 oral morphine equivalent (OME) or 15 tablets of 5 mg hydrocodone. Prescribing recommendations were posted all over the hospital in the perioperative areas and made into pocket-sized cards that were easily accessible for several months leading up to the start of the new legislative laws in July of 2018 regarding new recommendations for the number of opioids that an opioid-naive patient could be prescribed given a week's supply for an acute problem. Results from the 5722 patients in the preintervention phase demonstrated an overall mean ± standard deviation of OME prescribed during this period for all surgical procedures was 218.8 ± 113.7 (n = 722). In the postintervention phase, of the 129 subjects reviewed, the authors noted a significant decrease in mean OME prescribed by year (241.6 in 2015, 220.9 in 2016, 197.6 in 2017, and 71.9 in 2018; $P < .005$). In differentiating the preintervention to postintervention groups, it was noted that there was a 60% to 70% decrease in the average OME prescribed for each operation, which is statistically significant. This study demonstrated that using a standardized approach to multimodal pain management in the postoperative setting can greatly reduce the number of prescribed opioid prescriptions.

Additionally, researchers discussed how multimodal pain management[23] is readily available to providers and has strong evidence to support its efficacy. Providers must become knowledgeable about this type of pain management and how to use this approach effectively. They state that analgesics (eg, acetaminophen), NSAIDs, local anesthetics (eg, limb blocks and α_2-agonists), NMDA antagonists, and anticonvulsants are effective alternatives to using opioids alone. A meta-analysis study of 27 randomized clinical trials demonstrated no difference in postoperative bleeding between those groups who took ketorolac (33 of 1304 patients; 2.5%) and the control groups (21 of 1010; 2.1%) (odds ratio, 1.1; 95% confidence interval, 0.61–2.06; $P = .72$). Those postoperative colorectal patients on the enhanced recovery after surgery pathway who used a multimodal pain therapy approach were found to use 50% less opioids during their hospital stay, and most did not require opioids after discharge.

There continues to be a gap in continued education for multimodal pain management and provider narcotic prescribing methods. Providers must practice as patient advocates by continuously educating oneself on appropriate pain management therapies, especially because evidence-based practice is continuously evolving for better safe practices across the health care continuum.[24] For those new practicing providers in pain management, it is essential for health care institutions to provide core competency training during residency of future primary care providers, surgeons, and advanced practice providers. It is critical for providers to become aware of outpatient programs for opioid addiction and be able to provide access to those treatment programs or assist in getting the patient connected through the proper channels for access.

DISCUSSION

The opioid epidemic refers to a period in time around 2017 when the Department of Health and Human Services saw a surge in the amount of prescription opioids that were prescribed, which led to addiction, abuse, misuse, and even multiple deaths. A public health emergency was soon declared, with a plan put into place to combat the opioid crisis.[20] The world's largest consumer of opioids is the United States. The opioid epidemic has led to a public health crisis with increased rates of overdose and death and health care costs for medical facilities and patients, and has led to an increase in demand for first responders and the production of naloxone. Measures by health care providers must be taken to cut down on excessive overprescribing of opioids and continuing education on adequate pain management strategies, such as the benefits of multimodal therapies. Initiating a multimodal pain management approach, especially in the acute care setting, has proven to be beneficial with less opioid prescribing practices, opioid abuse, and deaths.[20]

Additionally, with the rise in opioid consumption comes an increase in emergency room visits, treatment admissions, and fatalities caused by overdose. Researchers reviewed several qualitative studies[25] on the progression from initial use of opioids to opioid abuse. A total of 2034 articles were evaluated and were screened for inclusion criteria for the review. The articles were narrowed down to 17 with the inclusion criteria of the population of the United States, prescription opioid abusers currently or previously before the study, studies with qualitative research methods, and participant quotes. The final inclusion criteria were motifs relating to prescription opioid abuse onset and the progression. There were numerous motivations for taking opioids. The participants stated "getting high" with the initial use of opioids made them continue to use the drugs. Furthermore, other motivations that participants reported were self-medicating physical pain, altering their mood, response to life stressors, or self-medicating psychological issues or even past trauma. A few other motivators discovered were enhanced sexual intimacy, boredom, heightened energy, the need to feel "normal," and self-blame. Understanding motivations and risk factors of the participants is imperative when deciding whether to prescribe or administer an opioid medication in a hospital setting, and when considering a multimodal approach to pain management. A vital component of pain management[24] in the acute setting is identifying patients with the greatest risk and provide them "opioid free anesthesia, and postoperative anesthesia." They further state this is accomplished by initiating a multimodal approach, such as regional anesthesia and lessening the dose and the time of the opioid prescription. Doing this allows prescribing different types of medications that work through differing mechanisms. The research also found opioid treatment in 10 days can lead to opioid dependence, and up to 15% of surgical patients can end up dependent on opioids following perioperative use. Statistics such as these continue to reinforce the recommendation of restricting opioids used during a perioperative time and encourages the benefits of a multimodal approach to pain relief. Lastly, research has found the multimodal approach that was most effective was the use of ketamine. The NMDA receptor plays a vital role in the central sensitization through the descending pathway by a nociceptive signal that is potentiated in the peripheral nervous system and is believed to play a role in inducing chronic and neuropathic pain. Even though methadone, dexamethasone, and magnesium all possess NMDA-blocking ability, ketamine has shown to be the leader for the perioperative approach. Furthermore, intranasal ketamine has been shown to be a safe and effective alternative to intranasal fentanyl, with the benefit of lowering use of opioids.

Additionally, there are more patients in the United States with chronic pain than cardiovascular disease. Opioids are often one of the options given to chronic pain patients. Patients on large amounts of opioids are a challenge for providers to manage in the outpatient setting, and in the perioperative setting. Because these patients may have an extreme tolerance to opioid medications, multimodal analgesia is remarkably important. Opioid-tolerant patients can have opioid-induced hyperalgesia (OIH), which is defined as having a state of enhanced nociceptive sensitization that comes when being exposed to opioids. Furthermore, OIH can also transpire in an acute setting, and with opioid-naive patients. An important adjunct to consider as a multimodal approach to postoperative pain management is dexmedetomidine. This drug is a powerful anxiolytic, and correspondingly provides opioid-sparing analgesic effects. According to a meta-analysis study in 2012, of the 1800 patients, only 39 participants received dexmedetomidine, which astonishingly revealed postoperative opioid consumption and pain intensity was markedly decreased.[26] The authors also discovered that dexmedetomidine was found to be a beneficial adjunct for management of OIH, especially in patients with substantial opioid tolerance and high opioid requirements.

SUMMARY

Research has demonstrated that multimodal pain management has been shown to reduce pain in the acute care setting and assists in developing chronic pain long term. When discussing multimodal pharmacologic measures in an around-the-clock fashion, it has been shown to remarkably decrease the need for opioid pain management therapy. More than 100 million people in the United States are suffering from chronic pain, and it is the primary cause of disability.[26] NSAIDs, such as ibuprofen, reduce opioid consumption by 25% to 30% and should be used as first-line therapy for those patients with mild to moderate pain, if given no contraindications. Acetaminophen, given that it is included in the NSAID class, does provide adequate analgesia to those with moderate to severe pain; however, it lacks anti-inflammatory properties. Its use has been proven effective if given conjunctively with other NSAIDs. NMDA antagonists, such as ketamine, are effective because they decrease central sensitization in acute and chronic pain, lowering pain hypersensitivity in the nociceptive pathways. Anticonvulsants, such as gabapentin and pregabalin, act as neuromodulators, decreasing neuronal excitability. Local anesthesia, such as single-shot blocks or continuous nerve blocks, helps to block the peripheral or central nerve pathways, and is thus a great option for perioperative and postoperative pain. Adequate pain management using a multimodal approach not only improves sleep, anxiety, mood, and the healing process but decreases opioid misuse and abuse, and proper use of health care resources.[24]

Furthermore, health care providers serve as patient advocates, and by practicing as a patient advocate, have a duty to protect patients by practicing safely and competently. Instituting a multimodal therapy approach through a combination of medications from different drug classes, such as acetaminophen, NSAIDs, local anesthetics (eg, limb blocks and α_2-agonists), NMDA antagonists, and anticonvulsants, helps target different pain receptors for better pain relief than using opioids alone. The multimodal approach assists in targeting various pain receptors to achieve adequate pain relief, thus using less opioids with a goal of less detrimental side effects. Multimodal drug therapy has proven to reduce the need for increased opioid usage, abuse, and mortalities while reducing hospital length of stay, costs, and use of resources for outpatient drug abuse treatment, thus bridging the gap between inappropriate opioid prescribing with prejudicial effects to safely and effectively control pain in the acute and chronic hospital setting.

CLINICS CARE POINTS

- Given the stricter state laws and regulations with the production of and prescribing of opioids, there still remains a gap in standardizing opioid prescribing practices.

- It is important to ascertain the need for opioids, especially in the acute care setting. Consumption of opioids for an extended period of time should warrant provider discussions to consider alternative medications, such as multimodal therapy, because this prevents unnecessary misuse and mortality.

- Multimodal pain management helps assist in targeting various pain receptors to achieve adequate pain control, thus lessening the prevalence of opioid misuse, abuse, and deaths.

- Instituting a multimodal therapy approach through a combination of medications from different drug classes, such as acetaminophen, NSAIDs, local anesthetics (eg, limb blocks and α_2-agonists), NMDA antagonists, and anticonvulsants, helps target different pain receptors for better pain relief than using opioids alone.

- Multimodal pain management assists in decreasing hospital length of stay, costs, and additional health care resources; increased patient satisfaction; and healthy lifestyle.
- Health care providers must practice as patient advocates in educating and re-educating themselves in appropriate pain management therapies, especially because evidence-based practice is continuously evolving for better safe practices across the health care continuum.

DISCLOSURE

The authors have nothing to disclose.

REFERENCES

1. Gabbey A. What is pain? Healthline 2021. Available at: https://www.healthline. com/health/pain#: ~ :text=Pain%20is%20a%20general%20term,stinging%2C% 20sore%2C%20and%20pinching.
2. Shipton EA, Shipton EE, Shipton A. A review of the opioid epidemic: what do we do about it? Pain Ther 2018;7(2018):23–36.
3. Manchikanti L, Singh V, Kaye A, et al. Lessons for better pain management in the future: learning from the past. Pain Ther 2020;9(2):373–91.
4. Graff V, Grosh T. Multimodal analgesia and alternatives to opioids for post-operative analgesia. J Anesth Patient Saf Found 2018;33(2):33–68.
5. American Nurses Association. Nursing's role in addressing nation's opioid crisis, . Nursing world. Available at:www.nursingworld.org.
6. Arnstein P. Multimodal approaches to pain management. Nursing 2011; 41(3):60–1.
7. Centers for Disease Control and Prevention. Chronic pain- United States, 2016. Morbidity and Mortality Weekly Report (MMWR) 2021;65(1):1–49. Opioid over-dose: understanding the epidemic.Available at: https://www.cdc.gov/ drugoverdose/epidemic/index.html.
8. Heins S, Frey K, Alexander C, et al. Reducing high-dose prescribing: state level morphine equivalent daily dose POLICIES, 2007-2017. Pain Med 2020;2(21): 308–16.
9. Skolnick P. The opioid epidemic: crisis and solutions. Annu Rev Pharmacol Tox-icol 2018;58:143–59.
10. Rauenzahn S, Del Fabbro E. Opioid management of pain: the impact of the pre-scription opioid abuse epidemic. Curr Opin Support Palliat Care 2014;3(8): 273–8.
11. Young A, Buvanendran A. Recent advances in multimodal analgesia. Anesthesi-ology Clin 2012;30(1):91–100.
12. London Pain Clinic. Multimodal analgesia. 2020. Available at:https://www. londonpainclinic.com/medication/multimodal-analgesia/. .
13. Hsu E. Medication overuse in chronic pain. Curr Pain Headache Rep 2017; 2(21):1–7.
14. Weigel D, Donovan K, Krug K, et al. Prescription opioid abuse and dependence: assessment strategies for counselors. J Couns Development 2007;85(2):211–5.
15. Thompson D. Doctors still overprescribing opioids in the U.S. WebMD. 2017. Available at:https://www.webmd.com/pain-management/news/20170731/ doctors-still-overprescribing-opioids-in-us#. .
16. National Safety Council. About the National Safety Council: workplace safety. 2021. Available at:https://www.nsc.org/company. .

17. Ng L, Cashman J. The management of acute pain. Medicine 2018;46(12):780–5.
18. National Institute of, Neurological Disorders and Stroke. Chronic pain information page. What research is being done?. 2021. Available at: www.ninds.nih.gov/Disorders/All-Disorders/Chronic-Pain-Information-Page.
19. Stanford Health Care. Management of pain without pain medications. 2021. Available at:https://stanfordhealthcare.org/medical-conditions/pain/pain/treatments/non-pharmacological-pain-management.html. .
20. U.S. Department of Health and Human Services. What is the U.S. opioid epidemic?. 2021. Available at:https://www.hhs.gov/opioids/about-the-epidemic/index.html. .
21. Dowell D, Haegerich T, Chou R. CDC guideline for prescribing opioids for chronic pain—United States, 2016. Morbidity Mortality Weekly Rep (MMWR) 2016; 65(1):1–49.
22. Zipple M, Braddock A. Success of hospital intervention and state legislation on decreasing and standardizing postoperative opioid prescribing practices. J Am Coll Surg 2018;229(2):158–63.
23. Wick E, Grant M, Wu C. Postoperative multimodal analgesia pain management with nonopioid analgesics and techniques: a review. JAMA Surg 2017;152(7): 691–7.
24. Wardhan, R., & Chelly, J. (2017). Recent advances in acute pain management: understanding the mechanisms of acute pain, the prescription of opioids, and the role of multimodal pain therapy. (6)2065.
25. Cicero T, Ellis M. The prescription opioid epidemic: a review of qualitative studies on the progression from initial use to abuse. Dialogues Clin Neurosci 2017;19(3): 259–69.
26. Patch R, Eldridge J, Pingree M. Dexmedetomidine as part of a multimodal analgesic treatment regimen for opioid hyperalgesia in a patient with significant opioid tolerance. Case Rep Anesthesiol 2017;2017(9876306):1–55.

The Role of Social Determinates of Health in Discharge Practices

Tamika Hudson, DNP, APRN, FNP-C

KEYWORDS

- Social determinants of health • Discharge planning • Discharge teaching • Nursing
- Health disparities

KEY POINTS

- Complex social constructs serve as barriers to health equity in postacute care settings.
- Nurses are ideally positioned to observe the changing needs associated with a patient's physical and social health status in preparation for discharge teaching and planning.
- Social determinants of health must be integrated into treatment and discharge planning to support positive health outcomes.

INTRODUCTION

The health and vitality of a community largely shape the mental, physical, and emotional health of its members. Environmental and social characteristics of a community may dictate quality and availability of education, food, health care, and safe dwellings. These conditions within the environment in which people are born, live, learn, work, play, worship, and age are described as social determinants of health (SDOH).[1] Health status and outcomes result from the intersectionality of economic stability, education, social and community context, health and health care, and neighborhood and built environment.[1] The influence of these conditions is evident before a patient ever presents to an acute care setting. Nurses must develop pertinent skills to assess how the social environment impacts patients' likelihood of a safe and healthy transition back into the community as they prepare patients for discharge.

Conventionally, major risks associated with inadequate discharge preparation and execution include medication errors, adverse drug events, and hospital readmissions.[2] These poor health outcomes can be compounded by complex social constructs that serve as barriers to health equity. MacNaughton-Doucet[3] attributed inadequate discharge execution to hospitals' task-oriented approach, which is dictated by medical diagnoses and an economic goal to recycle hospital beds. It is

Vanderbilt University, 461 21st Avenue South, Nashville, TN 37240, USA
E-mail address: tamika.s.hudson@vanderbilt.edu

Nurs Clin N Am 56 (2021) 369–378
https://doi.org/10.1016/j.cnur.2021.04.004
0029-6465/21/© 2021 Elsevier Inc. All rights reserved.

nursing.theclinics.com

commonplace for a patient's individualism, specifically socioeconomic factors, to be disregarded in a task-oriented and medically centric environment.[3] Thoughtful consideration of SDOH is paramount to minimize health disparities and promote health equity.

Nurses are often the first and last points of contact for patients in acute care settings. It can therefore be presumed that nurses establish and manage expectations for patient care and interactions during the hospital visit. Discharge preparation should occur throughout the hospitalization as a result of frequent assessment and monitoring of patient progress against expected outcomes.[4] Frequent and close patient-nurse interactions provide opportunities to observe the changing needs associated with a patient's physical and social health status.[4] The literature suggests recognition of best practices and standardization of discharge preparation. Advances in personalized medicine, clinical care, and pharmacology have excelled; however, there remains the necessity to better identify and characterize the SDOH that impact health outcomes.[2] Few studies underscore the importance of incorporating social determinants in processes to prepare patients for discharge planning and teaching. Identification of best practices for integrating SDOH into discharge planning and teaching is necessary for safe and culturally empathetic care (**Box 1**).

DISCHARGE PRACTICES
Discharge Planning

There are multiple dimensions to the discharge process. Discharge planning can be described as the development of discharge instructions to improve the efficiency and quality of health care delivery.[5] A foundational nursing text defined discharge planning as activities geared toward identifying proposed therapy and the need for additional resources before and after returning home.[6] Discharge planning has been considered the systematic organization of services to assist patients to self-manage after hospitalization.[3] Many of the instructions and resources referenced are aimed at a safe transition into the home environment; however, there are apparent variations in the methods nurses use to complete this task. Furthermore, a lack of consideration and integration of social determinants exists in preparing patients to return to the community. MacNaughton-Doucet[3] suggested this lack of evidence indicates a knowledge to practice gap of an essential component to patient care.

Preparation for discharge should occur upon arrival to the acute care setting and evolve over the course of the visit.[3,4,7] Potter and colleagues[6] suggested discharge

---

Box 1
Clinical care points for nurses

- Discharge practices should commence upon initial patient encounter.
- Nurse self-assessments and interventions for implicit bias are integral components of equitable patient care delivery related to discharge practices.
- Social determinants may be as impactful as physiologic influencers of health outcomes.
- Standardized approaches to discharged planning and teaching may be necessary to lessen knowledge to practice gaps.
- Interprofessional collaborative care and role delineation has been proven to enhance discharge practices.

Data from Refs.[2–4,7,22,23]

planning begin at initiation of care and include key family members. Morris and colleagues[8,9] conducted a review of the literature and concluded that 80% of nurses think discharge planning should begin upon patient admission despite associated studies indicating only 2% of an 8-hour nursing shift is dedicated to discharge planning. The initial patient admissions interview typically obtained by the nurse provides integral data to assist in proper planning for activities within the clinical setting and on discharge. This interview provides historical context relative to the patient's current condition. External influences on health should be critically assessed with similar scrutiny as internal and physiologic indicators. The nursing care plan constructed after the initial interview can serve as a road map for favorable health outcomes by analyzing the patient holistically. Care plans provide valuable information, including nursing diagnoses, expected outcomes, and interventions.[6]

Nurses must think beyond medical management to ensure equitable and inclusive nursing practices. MacNaughton-Doucet[3] attested that hospital-based nurses that have not worked in the community may have difficulty anticipating socioeconomic issues in the safety and predictability of the hospital setting.[3] The investigator also reported barriers to effective discharge planning include absence of continuity of care, role confusion, lack of an interprofessional team, competing priorities, and power dynamics.[3] In addition, there is a lack of nationally approved evidence-based practice tools to assist in the planning of transitional care despite the vast amount of discharge decisions made per year.[10] These findings underscore the importance of identifying best practices to ensure positive health outcomes for patients.

A Cochrane Review examined 24 randomized controlled trials consisting of 8098 participants to identify best practices for discharging patients home from the acute care setting.[5] The review surmised that personalized discharge plans can encourage reductions in the length of stay in acute care settings and readmission rates when compared with standard discharge planning.[5] This finding is of particular importance considering acute care settings with excess readmissions receive financial penalties that include a reduction or elimination of reimbursement for readmitted patients.[11] Elderly individuals and people of color are at an even higher risk of readmission because of societal constructs and determinants.[2]

The landscape of our current society is calling for a more inclusive approach to social and civic engagement. Nurses, as other health care professionals, are charged with ensuring all members of our society receive inclusive and equitable care. An emphasis on collaborative care and role delineation has been proven to enhance discharge practices. The lack of clear role delineation for discharge teaching, specifically, can result in duplication, omission, inconsistencies, and poor adherence to teachings.[4]

Weiss and colleagues[4] surmised the clinical nurse is central and continuous throughout hospitalization, thus the discharge process; however, other members of the clinical team have specific roles and responsibilities and should be held accountable in the discharge process. MacNaughton-Doucet[3] had similar findings, asserting that the interdisciplinary team is responsible for a seamless transition home from the acute care environment because of a more comprehensive outlook on problem solving and approaches to patient-centered care.[3] When assessing opinions of health care professionals, 44% of study participants reported feeling that there was inadequate staffing on the discharge team; 66% of participants thought the discharge team could benefit from additional training, and 80% thought administrative requirements regarding length of stay resulted in inadequate and expedited discharge planning.[3]

Discharge Teaching

Discharge teaching is a fundamental component of discharge practices. Although the concepts of discharge planning and discharge teaching are intertwined, terminology should not be used interchangeably. Discharge teaching is the collective educational intervention occurring during hospitalization to prepare the patient and family to transition back into the community.[4] Discharge teaching should occur in tandem with other discharge planning and practice efforts.

Content for discharge teaching typically includes review of the health condition, test results, follow-up appointments, instructions for safe care, current medications, warning signs for symptom worsening, and contact information for the primary care provider.[4] The goal of the educational intervention is to provide adequate information to make informed decisions and enhance skills and confidence for postacute care.[4] Social determinants should influence educational planning and teaching strategies. Optimal discharge practices occur where discharge planning, teaching, and coordination intersect.

SOCIAL DETERMINANTS OF HEALTH

The Office of Disease Prevention and Health Prevention consider the presence of poverty, inadequate housing, a lack of food, and unemployment effective gauges of economic stability within a community.[1] Similarly, the neighborhood and built environment are predicated on the quality of housing structures, food accessibility, crime and violence rates, and environmental conditions, such as mold, clean drinking water, and cigarette smoke. The lack of financial resources to secure safe housing and obtain healthy food options is another threat to the health and well-being of community members. **Table 1** identifies social determinants that impact discharge practices.

Table 1	
Examples of social determinants that impact discharge planning and teaching	
Economic stability	Employment status
	Food insecurity
	Occupational hazards
	Poverty
	Transportation
Education	Educational attainment
	Illiteracy
	Language barriers
Social and community context	Discrimination
	Health disparities
	Implicit bias
	Racism
Health and health care	Adherence to follow-up appointments
	Health insurance status
	Health literacy
	Lifestyle choices
	Medication regimen
	Weathering secondary to chronic oppression
Neighborhood and built environment	Crime
	Inadequate social or physical infrastructure
	Inappropriate or lack of transitional care

Data from Refs.[1–3,7,12–17,19,20,22,24]

Research suggests the time frame immediately upon discharge is a vulnerable time for patients.[2] Therefore, it is critically important that nurses consider elements beyond traditional medically oriented questions when assessing for barriers to self-care. Tubbs-Cooley and colleagues[7] found that children not categorized as having a high medical complexity reported difficulties obtaining follow-up appointments and services. A key component of assessing SDOH includes asking sensitive questions pertaining to lifestyle, home environment, and finances.[12] MacNaughton-Doucet[3] agreed that asking questions about SDOH may provide solutions to narrow the knowledge to practice gap between patient needs and accessibility of resources.

Economic Stability

Employment, food security, housing, and affluence are drivers of economic stability.[1] The converse can inhibit the ability to foster an environment for individuals to thrive economically. Poverty is a deprivation concern that can have severe physical and mental consequences that often lead to comorbidities.[13] Nurses can examine a patient's economic stability by inquiring about the presence and nature of employment. Certain professions may place vulnerable patients at an increased risk of worsening symptoms requiring readmission to the acute care setting. Occupational environments that require physically rigorous tasks or involve toxins and pollutants should influence content presented during discharge planning and teaching. In addition, knowledge of the full nature of employment will encourage dialogue regarding favorable scheduling of follow-up appointments after discharge.

Economic standing to secure healthy meals directly impacts health and wellness. In 2019, 13.6% of households in the United States were food insecure.[14] Individuals who identified as food insecure were more likely to report ill health and an inability to pay for housing and utilities.[3] Inquiring about current food intake routines and practices should be incorporated into patient interviews. Patients residing in food deserts may have limited availability of healthy food options to comply with suggestions provided during discharge teaching. Similarly, medications required to be taken with meals may be avoided if a patient has limited financial resources to secure food or the medications themselves. It is imperative that, as intuitively the nurse conducts a physical assessment to identify deviations outside of expected physical assessment findings, the nurse should also seek to discover social barriers to optimal health.

The Hunger Vital Sign was developed by Drs Erin Hager and Anna Quigg in 2010 to measure food security.[12] Families are considered at risk for food insecurity if they answer, "often true" or "sometimes true" to the following questions: "Within the past 12 months we worried whether our food would run out before we got money to buy more" and/or "Within the past 12 months the food we bought just didn't last and we didn't have money to get more."[12] This measurement tool can be instrumental in identifying the need for resources to supply and support nutrition for patients and family members.

Lack of transportation may also be an indicator of economic instability. It is important that nurses inquire about transportation plans for activities prescribed in post-discharge instructions. Patients that are unable to present for diagnostic testing, rehabilitation services, follow-up appointments, or other postacute plans cannot fully benefit from the regimens designed to support recovery. The significance of a lack of transportation extends beyond possession of a vehicle. Considerations and discussions regarding reliable transportation to postacute follow-up services should be made relative to distance to bus stops, number of bus transfers, total travel time, safe bus stop locations, and insurance coverage for transportation services.[12] Similar attention is required for investigating processes to acquire medication as needed.

Population-specific concerns may present for patients residing in rural areas. Nurses should consider additional fuel costs for diagnostic services and specialty care outside of the patient's immediate environment.[12]

Education

Educational attainment, language, and literacy are associated with the education domain of social determinants. Individuals with limited education often have poorer health outcomes. Cafagna and Seghieri[15] concluded that patients recently diagnosed with an acute myocardial infarction and limited education were more likely to die within 30 days of being discharged from the acute care setting. That finding was consistent with existing evidence indicating higher rates of death for less educated patients despite efforts to promote quality health care and access for all patients.[15] The knowledge to practice gap related to social determinants has dire effects, including death. Low educational attainment has been associated with poor self-management likely because of an unawareness of symptom severity, and consequently, an inability to transfer instructions into practice, adhere to medication regimens, or obtain follow-up care.[15]

Language barriers impede information gathering and patient-centered goal setting for discharge practices. Patients presenting to the acute care setting with cultural backgrounds that differ from the nurse may have contrasting perceptions and expectations regarding utilization of the health care system.[16] An inability to communicate effectively with a patient hinders the ability to ascertain this valuable information and can negatively impact trust and relationship building. Mistrust paired with language barriers can cause ethnically underrepresented populations to seek shorter hospital stays, which may directly impact access to necessary services, such as rehabilitation.[16] Consequently, utilization of interpreters and language lines should be standard practice as available. Similarly, printed materials must be provided to the patient in their preferred language as available. These practices are culturally empathetic and foster inclusivity.

Verbal and written communication of discharge planning and teaching is vitally important to positive health outcomes after discharge. A patient's ability to understand verbal and written materials should be established as an element of discharge practices. The most fundamental definition of being literate is the ability to read and write.[17] The International Literacy Association described literacy as the "ability to identify, understand, interpret, create, compute, and communicate using visual, audible, and digital materials across disciplines and in any context".[18] With 21% of American adults considered illiterate or functionally illiterate in 2019, nurses must evaluate the way in which information is conveyed to patients.[19] The nurse should also ensure the print is large enough for patients with visual impairment and provide braille as needed and available.

Social and Community Context

Racism, discrimination, and implicit bias provide social and community context for SDOH. Health care inaccessibility for ethnically underrepresented individuals is recognized as a global challenge.[16] Inequity as a result of racism drives health disparities and poor health outcomes across the life span.[20] Disproportionate levels of preterm birth and infant mortality in black and Latinx communities demonstrate that even the youngest members of our society are impacted by systemic racism and structural inequities. In recognition, the American Academy of Pediatrics authored guidelines for high-risk newborns inclusive of risk identification, discharge timing, and post-discharge care.[20,21] An emphasis was placed on discharge planning that focuses on parental education, routine health care, care planning for complex health conditions, comprehensive home care, identification and involvement of support services, and designation of follow-up care.[20,21] Preterm birth and infant mortality are merely examples of detrimental conditions that can benefit from comprehensive discharge management.

The existence of racism in the clinical environment rarely presents explicitly; rather, it is more commonly exhibited as implicit bias. Implicit bias is recognized as the "attitudes or stereotypes that affect our understanding, actions, and decisions in an unconscious manner."[22] In the clinical environment, implicit basis has resulted in fewer prescriptions for pain medication, fewer medically indicated bypass surgeries, decreased recommendations for dialysis or kidney transplantation, and increased recommendations for lower limb amputations secondary to diabetes.[23] Implicit bias informs every aspect of patient care, including discharge practices. Biases are often a result of perceptions regarding race and perceived socioeconomic status.

Decisions regarding transitional care and the selection of treatment modalities are prime examples of where bias presents in discharge practices. Transitional care is a broad term for interventions that facilitate safe and timely transfer of patients between levels of care and settings.[24] This care model encompasses discharges within institutions, outside facilities, and to the communities with expected follow-up care with primary care providers. Assessment and recognition of insurance coverage, social support, identification with specific vulnerable patient populations, and other external drivers are required for effective coordination of discharge efforts. Recognition of biases that dictate planning should be prioritized in the safe transition of patient.

Table 2 illustrates tools to assist nurses in identifying and addressing bias. Project Implicit, sponsored by Harvard University, created the Implicit Association Test to assist in identifying and measuring attitudes and stereotypes.[25] The EveryONE Project from the American Academy of Family Physicians created an implicit basis training guide to identify and reduce implicit bias in clinical practice.[26] Last, individuals seeking to rid themselves of bias can participate in a 7-day cleanse created by the Kirwan Institute.[22] The removal of assumptions allow the nurse to enter the planning process with uncorrupted intentions and a readiness to support the whole patient.

Health and Health Care

Although the availability and provision of health insurance can serve as a predictor for positive health outcomes, it should not be considered a sole indicator. In the United States, Medicaid beneficiaries consistently have poor health outcomes.[27] Specifically, studies demonstrate Medicaid beneficiaries have more complications despite being higher utilizers of resources when compared with patients with private insurance.[27] The Medicaid population is more likely to undergo major surgery, have higher risks

Table 2	
Tools for implicit bias assessment and amelioration	
EveryONE Project	The EveryONE project created an Implicit Bias Training guide to promote awareness of implicit bias and provide resources for health care professionals to reduce its negative effects on patients. https://www.aafp.org/news/practice-professional-issues/20200115implicitbias.html
Implicit Association Test	The Implicit Association Test measures associations between concepts and stereotypes. https://implicit.harvard.edu/implicit/takeatest.html

Data from Refs.[25,26]

of wound complications, and have higher in-hospital mortality, which may be in part attributed to having more comorbidities and being more likely to smoke.[27] Lifestyle choices, poverty, and societal inequities may be more significant in this paradigm than the existence of one or more health conditions. Weathering secondary to chronic oppression can be experienced by populations with limited financial resources. Nurses should recognize that patients with low socioeconomic status have additional risk factors that necessitate comprehensive discharge practices.

Health literacy is a component of the health and health care domain of SDOH that significantly impacts how patients navigate the health care system. It has rudimentary implications for discharge planning and teaching. Health literacy differs somewhat from literacy previously mentioned. Health literacy describes the "capacity to obtain, process, and understand basic health information needed to make appropriate health decisions."[28]

Meyers and colleagues[2] highlighted important relationships between health literacy and medication adherence, keeping follow-up appointments, and recognition of side effects and appropriate next steps should side effects present. The investigators also surmised that low health literacy was associated with hospital readmission and mortality,[2] which is of particular importance because it is most common in vulnerable populations. Elderly, ethnically underrepresented, medically underserved, and individuals with low socioeconomic status tend to have a higher prevalence of low health literacy. Adini[16] attested that access and equity to posthospital care is in part dependent on enhanced health literacy and health education for all sectors of our society.

Neighborhood and Built Environment

One of the most critical decisions to be made by the patient, family, and clinicians is the location to which the patient will be discharged. A collaborative approach to decision making is most effective in aligning patient desires with appropriate medical oversight. Although an immediate outcome goal of discharge preparation is discharge readiness, intermediate goals are associated with successful patient and family management of patient needs in the outpatient setting or appropriate transfer to a postacute environment for continuation of treatment.[4]

Environmental conditions are important SDOH characteristics within the neighborhood and built environment domain that require careful consideration. Assessment of social and physical infrastructures that the patient will transition or return to is integral to planning efforts. The presence of crime or lack of social support is as important as the presence of stairs or other potential barriers to safety and well-being. Innovative approaches are required to ensure goals are met for each stakeholder.

It can be challenging to coordinate discharge processes while confirming the quality of services provided by other health care entities. The referring clinical team, including the nurse, has a responsibility to investigate safe and competent care of transitional care providers before patient discharge. Burke and Ibrahim[29] concluded that clinicians may face pressures in making discharge decisions quickly, leading them to select a skilled nursing facility (SNF) over the home. Weiss and colleagues[4] agreed, proclaiming discharge teaching and decision making left until the day of discharge decrease patient attentiveness and nurse effectiveness, becoming problematic when there is variability in quality of care that can influence health outcomes. Black patients who underwent joint arthroplasty were more likely to be discharged to an SNF in comparison to their white counterparts who were more likely to be discharged to the home environment.[29] This finding is of critical importance considering blacks have a higher probability of receiving care at lower-quality SNF because of proximity, therefore increasing the risk for poor outcomes and enhanced disparities.[29]

The investigators provided evidence to support that home care leads to similar recovery outcomes as institutional postacute care after joint replacement at significantly lower costs.[29] A study conducted by Tubbs-Cooley and colleagues[7] revealed nurse home visiting programs can address SDOH and reduce disparities by minimizing preventable injuries and assisting in disease management. Specifically, study findings support home visit interventions for establishing follow-up care after discharge, enhancing medication management, and monitoring physiologic status changes for pediatric patients.[7]

SUMMARY

Societal and cultural influences are calling for more inclusive approaches to civic engagement. The health care industry serves as an integral component of this emphasis. Recognition and consideration of SDOH are critical to minimizing health disparities, enhancing health equity, and supporting positive patient outcomes. Nurses are key drivers in the course of patient treatment in acute care settings. Initiating discharge practices on admission enable nurses to assess patient readiness for discharge and plan for safe transfer to the community or other recommended medical facility for continuation of care. In the prioritization for inclusive care for all, social factors must be examined with similar fervor as physiologic presentations in the acute care environment.

DISCLOSURE

The author has nothing to disclose.

REFERENCES

1. Office of Disease Prevention and Health Prevention. Social determinants of health. 2020. Available at: https://www.healthypeople.gov/2020/topics-objectives/topic/social-determinants-of-health. Accessed December 15, 2020.
2. Meyers AG, Salanitro A, Wallston KA, et al. Determinants of health after hospitalization discharge: rationale and design of the Vanderbilt Inpatient Cohort Study (VICS). BMC Health Serv Res 2014;14:1–10.
3. MacNaughton-Doucet LJ. Determinants of health in discharge planning for seniors: asking the right questions. Can J Aging 2013;32:307–14.
4. Weiss ME, Bobay K, Bahr SJ, et al. A model for hospital discharge preparation: from case management to care transition. J Nurs Mang 2015;45:606–14.
5. An D. Cochrane Review Brief: discharge planning from the hospital to home. Online J Issues Nurs 2014;20. https://doi.org/10.3912/OJIN.Vol20No02CRBCol01.
6. Potter PA, Perry AG, Hall A, et al. Fundamentals of nursing. St Louis: Mosby Elsevier; 2017. p. 1311.
7. Tubbs-Cooley HL, Riddle SW, Gold JM, et al. Paediatric clinical and social concerns identified by home visit nurses in the immediate post discharge period. J Adv Nurs 2020;76:1394–403.
8. Morris J, Winfield L, Young K. Registered nurses' perceptions of the discharge planning process for adult patients in an acute hospital. J Nurs Educ Prac 2012;2:28–38.
9. Hayajneh AA, Hweidi IM, Abu Dieh MW. Nurses' knowledge, perception, and practice toward discharge planning in acute care settings: a systematic review. Nurs Open 2020;7:1313–20.
10. Bowles KH, Chittams J, Heil E, et al. Successful electronic implementation of discharge referral decision support has a positive impact on 30- and 60-day readmissions. Res Nurs Health 2015;38:102–14.

11. Patel PR, Bechman S. Discharge planning. Treasure Island, FL. 2020. Available at: https://www.ncbi.nlm.nih.gov/books/NBK557819/. Accessed December 18, 2021.

12. Bruner E. Social determinants of health: the zip code is the most important number on the patient's chart! Virginia Nurses Today 2020;28:12–9.

13. Duncan M. Population health management and its relevance to community nurses. Br J Community Nurs 2019;24:596–9.

14. United States Department of Agriculture. Food security in the U.S. In: Economic Research Service. 2020. Available at: https://www.ers.usda.gov/topics/food-nutrition-assistance/food-security-in-the-us/key-statistics-graphics.aspx. Accessed December 18, 2020.

15. Cafagna G, Seghieri C. Educational level and 30-day outcomes after hospitalization for acute myocardial infarction in Italy. BMC Health Serv Res 2017;17:1–11.

16. Adini B. Ethnic inequality within the elderly population in utilizing healthcare services. Isr J Health Policy Res 2019;8:1–4.

17. Merriam-Webster. Literacy. Available at: https://www.merriam-webster.com/dictionary/literate. Accessed December 19, 2020.

18. International Literacy Association. Why literacy? 2020. Available at: https://www.literacyworldwide.org/about-us/why-literacy. Accessed December 19, 2020.

19. National Center for Educational Statistics. Adult literacy in the United States. In: Data Points, U.S. Department of Education NCES. 2019. Available at: https://nces.ed.gov/datapoints/2019179.asp. Accessed December 19, 2020.

20. Beck AF, Edwards EM, Horbar JD, et al. The color of health: how racism, segregation, and inequality affect the health and well-being of preterm infants and their families. Pediatr Res 2020;87:227–34.

21. American Academy of Pediatrics Committee on Fetus and Newborn. Hospital discharge of the high-risk neonate. Pediatrics 2008;122:119–1126.

22. The Kirwan Institute for the Study of Race and Ethnicity. Understanding implicit bias. 2015. Available at: http://kirwaninstitute.osu.edu/research/understanding-implicit-bias/. Accessed December 19, 2020.

23. American Academy of Family Physicians. Addressing implicit bias in health care delivery. In Implicit Bias. 2020. Available at: https://www.aafp.org/about/policies/all/implicit-bias.html. Accessed December 19, 2020.

24. Allen J, Hutchinson AM, Brown R, et al. Quality care outcomes following transitional care interventions for older people from hospital to home: a systematic review. BMC Health Serv Res 2014;14:1–18.

25. Project Implicit. The Implicit Association Test. 2011. Available at: https://implicit.harvard.edu/implicit/takeatest.html. Accessed December 19, 2020.

26. Crawford C. The EveryONE Project unveils implicit basis training guide. In: AAFP Practice and Career. 2020. Available at: https://www.aafp.org/news/practice-professional-issues/20200115implicitbias.html. Accessed December 19, 2020.

27. Clafttin J, Dimick JB, Campbell DA, et al. Understanding disparities in surgical outcomes for Medicaid beneficiaries. World J Surg 2019;43:981–7.

28. Human Resources and Services Administration. Health literacy. 2019. Available at: https://www.hrsa.gov/about/organization/bureaus/ohe/health-literacy/index.html#:~:text=Health%20literacy%20is%20the%20degree,Minority%20poppopulati. Accessed December 19, 2020.

29. Burke RE, Ibrahim SA. Discharge destination and disparities in postoperative care. JAMA 2018;319:1653–4.

Basic Airway Management for the Professional Nurse

Denise H. Tola, DNP, CRNA, CHSE[a],*, Alyssa Rojo, MSN, RN[b], Brett Morgan, DNP, CRNA[b]

KEYWORDS

- Basic airway management • RN generalist • Oxygen delivery systems
- Respiratory failure

KEY POINTS

- Recognize respiratory deterioration.
- Distinguish various oxygen delivery systems and the advantages and disadvantages of each.
- Review basic airway management: opening the airway, adjunct airway equipment, and techniques for use.
- Equipment needed for emergency airway management.

INTRODUCTION

The registered nurse (RN) generalist is pivotal to the care of a patient with the signs of impending respiratory failure. The RN must be competent in the recognition of the signs of respiratory compromise and possess the confidence to intervene appropriately and without delay. This article reviews the signs of respiratory deterioration, the physical assessment of the patient experiencing respiratory distress, and respiratory laboratory studies. Modes of oxygen therapy, basic airway management techniques, including bag mask ventilation (BMV), and use of oropharyngeal and nasopharyngeal airways are also discussed. Preparation for intubation of the trachea, equipment to be assembled, and medications frequently used for intubation are outlined. The scope of practice for the RN generalist may not include advanced airway management, but in the interest of patient safety, they should be familiar with procedures and equipment to facilitate efficient airway intervention.

The authors have nothing to disclose.
^a Nurse Anesthesia Program, Duke University School of Nursing, 307 Trent Drive, Durham, NC 27710, USA; ^b American Association of Nurse Anesthetists, 222 South Prospect Avenue, Park Ridge, IL 60068, USA
* Corresponding author.
E-mail address: Denise.tola@duke.edu

Nurs Clin N Am 56 (2021) 379–388
https://doi.org/10.1016/j.cnur.2021.04.005
0029-6465/21/© 2021 Elsevier Inc. All rights reserved.

DISCUSSION
Identifying Respiratory Failure or Airway Compromise

Nurses are often the first personnel to identify a patient experiencing airway distress. It is therefore essential that all nursing staff be familiar with the basic signs and symptoms of respiratory deterioration and airway compromise. In addition, understanding common airway and respiratory assessment techniques and tools will equip nurses with additional methods for identifying patients in crisis earlier before irreversible harm has been caused.[1]

There are 2 major types of respiratory failure. The first is known as hypoxemic respiratory failure, which results from lung failure.[2] The second is known as hypercapnic failure, which results from mechanical failure of the pulmonary system.[2] **Table 1** presents common signs and symptoms of hypoxemic and hypercapnic respiratory failure.[2]

Patient assessment

A thorough patient examination is critical in identifying patients who need emergency intervention because of respiratory failure. The initial assessment should focus on 3 factors: vital signs, work of breathing, and level of consciousness.[3] These factors will provide the information needed to determine if a patient is in crisis.[3]

A patient's vital signs may provide some of the most useful information in identifying respiratory failure and determining its severity. An increase in respiratory rate, tachypnea, is one of the earliest compensatory responses to respiratory failure.[4] It is not until the very late stages of hypercapnic failure that patients begin to slow down their breathing.[4] Initially, patients may also exhibit a high pulse rate and their blood pressure may be elevated[4]; this is also a compensatory response intended to increase the delivery of oxygen to the body's tissues. Once the body is no longer able to compensate, patients can exhibit bradycardia and low blood pressure.[4] Finally, blood oxygen saturation, estimated by a pulse oximeter, provides an estimation of the saturation of a patient's hemoglobin with oxygen.[5] A pulse oximeter reading of 90% corresponds with Pao_2 of 60 mm Hg.[5]

The physical examination should initially focus on assessing the patient's work of breathing. Patients should be monitored for tachypnea, keeping in mind age-specific norms (**Table 2**).[6] When tachypnea is accompanied by respiratory muscle retraction, nasal flaring, or additional sounds of increased work, such as grunting, intervention to support the patient or prevent respiratory collapse is often necessary.[2]

Table 1	
Signs and symptoms of respiratory failure	
Hypoxic Respiratory Failure	**Hypercapnic Respiratory Failure**
Mild to moderate	Mild to moderate
• Dyspnea	• Dyspnea
• Pallor	• Reduced reflexes
• Hypertension	• Flushing
• Disorientation or euphoria	• Tachypnea
• Euphoria	• Tachycardia
• Tachycardia	• Drowsiness or confusion
Severe	Severe
• Bradycardia	• Coma
• Cyanosis	• Papilledema
• Hypotension	
• Seizures	

Table 2 General respiratory rate by age	
Age Range	**Breaths/min**
Newborns-infants	30–60
Toddlers	24–30
Children	12–30
Adults	8–20

Patients should also be monitored for slow or shallow breathing. Breathing slower than normal, bradypnea, is often seen in patients with neuromuscular disorders or patients experiencing respiratory center failure.[2] When resulting from a neuromuscular compromise, patients may also demonstrate shallow, nonlabored breathing patterns.[2] Along with respiratory rate, the symmetry of chest wall expansion should also be observed. Patients experiencing severe respiratory distress may exhibit paradoxic movement of the chest and abdomen, and asymmetric chest wall expansion could indicate significant lung injury or pathologic condition.[2]

Although the physical assessment will focus primarily on the respiratory system, a compromised airway and respiratory failure can also result from issues found in other body systems. For instance, it is important to assess the cardiovascular system to eliminate conditions, such as heart failure or arrhythmias, as the cause of breathing issues.[2] Mental status changes can also originate as both symptoms of respiratory compromise and neurologic impairment.[2] Using assessment tools, such as the Glasgow Coma Scale (GCS), allows nurses to assess patients for severe neurologic compromise.[7] A GSC score of 8 or lower indicates severe impairment that is likely to interfere with a patient's ability to control his or her airway secretions.[7] Experts recommend tracheal intubation for these patients.[7]

Diagnostic testing

Diagnostic testing is useful in determining both the origin of respiratory distress and the severity. Chest radiographs should be performed in all patients experiencing respiratory failure, and if a cardiac origin is suspected, an electrocardiogram and echocardiogram may be warranted.[2] Common laboratory studies performed to assess the respiratory status are the arterial blood gas (ABG), complete blood count with differential (CBC), and a comprehensive metabolic panel.[2] It is important to note that although these tests are very useful, emergency interventions should not be delayed awaiting their results.[2]

The ABG accurately evaluates a patient's ability to exchange oxygen and carbon dioxide and provides insight into the type and duration of respiratory failure.[8,9] The 3 major components of an ABG are pH, $Paco_2$, and Hco_3.[8,9] Nurses should examine the pH to determine if the patient is in the normal range (7.35–7.45), above or alkalotic (>7.45), or below or acidotic (<7.35).[8] The $Paco_2$ is useful in determining the origin of the respiratory failure, either respiratory or metabolic.[9] The final factor is Hco_3, which allows the nurse to fully evaluate the ABG.[9] ABG interpretation requires additional training and experience; however, all nurses should be able to identify key components and abnormalities requiring further expert interpretation and intervention when appropriate.[8]

Additional blood tests are also useful in determining the cause of respiratory failure. The CBC provides insight into causes, such as infection, as well as allows nurses to assess for conditions that decrease the blood's ability to carry oxygen, such as anemia.[2] Metabolic panels are also useful, as they may help to identify the causes of conditions contributing to respiratory failure; for example, electrolyte abnormalities, such as low sodium, which can cause seizures and neurologic compromise.[2]

Oxygen Delivery Systems

There are various modes of oxygen delivery to choose from when deciding which type of delivery system is the best for the patient. This decision is made based on the patient's diagnosis, their oxygen requirement, ease and efficacy of application, as well as the patient's acceptance.[10] It is important to understand the oxygen flow rate as well as the fraction of inspired oxygen percentage (Fio_2). The oxygen flow rate is the *amount* of oxygen (in L/min) the patient inhales, whereas the Fio_2 is the *percentage of oxygen concentration* the patient inhales.[11] Depending on the type of oxygen delivery system used, the percentage of oxygen inhaled is often inexact.[11] For example, room air contains 21% oxygen, so the Fio_2 of room air is 21%.[11] **Table 3** provides additional information on specific oxygen delivery systems.

Categorizing oxygen devices

Oxygen devices can be categorized into 3 types: Low flow, reservoir, and high flow[10]:

- Low-flow oxygen delivery systems are diluted with room air, as they alone provide a flow rate that is lower than what the patient's inspiratory needs are.[12]
  ○ Common low-flow devices include a low-flow nasal cannula, non-rebreather mask, and a transtracheal oxygen catheter.[12]
- Reservoir systems store oxygen during the patient's inspiration and expiration by using a reservoir device.[10] As oxygen is not wasted, these can be viewed as a more efficient process.[10]
  ○ Common reservoir devices are reservoir cannulas and reservoir masks.[10]
- High-flow delivery systems supply oxygen higher than the patient's inspiratory needs, which allows a precise Fio_2 to be chosen.[10]
  ○ Common high-flow devices are the rebreather mask, simple face mask, Venturi mask, and the high-flow nasal cannula.[12]

Oxygen storage

Hospitals may store oxygen in varying ways to be available in all, or most, patient rooms. The most common method hospitals use is to have large tanks of liquid oxygen (LOX) on site.[13] This method is the most efficient, as 1 L of LOX equals approximately 860 L of gaseous oxygen.[13] One of the alternatives is to use compressed gas cylinders, which are often used during patient transport or as a quick replacement during an LOX disruption.[13] E cylinders are smaller with approximately 679 L of oxygen and are used for short-term patient transport.[13] H cylinders are larger with approximately 6900 L of oxygen and can be used for a longer length of time.[13] Although compressed gas cylinders are effective, and often necessary, in certain situations, using an LOX system is much safer for patients and staff.

Although both systems must be kept away from flammable material, the internal pressure, otherwise known as psi, is vastly different between the storage systems.[13] Knowing the approximate psi of the oxygen storage system and appropriate handling of cylinders is particularly important, as it relates directly to patient and clinician safety. The LOX system's psi is approximately 130 psi, whereas compressed gas E cylinders contain 2000 to 2200 psi.[13] Compressed gas cylinders can turn into destructive projectiles if mishandled.

Oxygen delivery systems explained

Five of the most commonly used oxygen delivery systems that the nurse may encounter are the low- and high-flow nasal cannula, simple face mask, Venturi

Table 3
Types of oxygen delivery systems and characteristics[10,12,14]

Type of Oxygen Delivery	Flow Rates	Fio₂	Clinical Considerations	Notes
Low-flow nasal cannula	1–6 L/min	24%–44%	• Used for mild hypoxia • Avoid an oxygen flow of >6 L/min, as it can dry the nasal mucosa • Not to be used in patients who have deviated septum or nasal polyps	Most commonly used, as the patient is able to talk and eat while wearing
Simple face mask	5–10 L/min	35%–55%	• Used when a moderate amount of oxygen is needed • Humidified air may be added if patient experiences nasal mucosa dryness	Some patients may feel claustrophobic with the mask on, as eating and drinking may be difficult
Non-rebreather	10–15 L/min	Up to 90%	• Best used in a cardiopulmonary emergency with severely hypoxic patients • Increases risk for carbon dioxide retention and aspiration from vomiting • Oxygen flow <10 L/min can cause the bag to collapse during inspiration	Wearing this is uncomfortable and drying, as the mask must fit tightly to the face
Venturi mask	Dependent on the port chosen	24%–50%	• Frequently used with chronic obstructive pulmonary disease patients • Allows exact Fio₂ measurement with the use of different color-coded sized ports	Not drying to the mucous membranes yet can hinder talking and eating
High-flow nasal cannula	Up to 60 L/min	Up to 100%	• Air is heated and humidified • Reduces the work of breathing, as the high flow and increased humidity allows secretions to be cleared • Associated with decreased mouth discomfort and increased overall comfort	A very comfortable option for many patients

mask, and the non-rebreather. **Table 3** describes each oxygen delivery system and important information to note to best care for the patient holistically.[10,12,14]

Basic Airway Management Techniques

Most health care clinicians are required to maintain their basic life support skills, which includes basic airway management. The RN generalist, however, may not have the opportunity to use or practice basic airway management skills on a regular basis. Therefore, review of the basics may be helpful. Opening the airway is the first step if a patient is found to be unconscious.[15] This step alone may indeed stimulate respiratory effort if the cause was obstruction from the tongue. There are 2 main techniques for opening the airway.[16] The first is the simple head tilt, chin lift.[16] This maneuver is performed by applying one hand to the patient's forehead to tilt the head back slightly while the other hand pulls the chin up.[16] The head tilt will usually open the airway while the chin lift will often move the tongue forward as the mandible is displaced, thus alleviating tongue obstruction.[16] The second technique is the jaw thrust maneuver.[16] The jaw thrust maneuver is performed by placing both hands at the sides of the patient's head at the mandibular angles.[16] With the thumbs pointing toward the feet, the index and middle fingers push the mandible forward while the thumbs can gently apply pressure to the chin to open the airway.[16] The jaw thrust should be used if there is suspected or known cervical injury.[16]

Adjunct airway equipment

BMV may be required if the patient does not spontaneously breathe after opening the airway or if the respiratory effort is insufficient to produce adequate ventilation. The efficiency of BMV requires an open patent airway, an adequate mask seal, and the generation of enough pressure to produce chest rise with compression of the bag.[16,17] A one-person technique can be difficult for the inexperienced. Usually, the left hand is used to form a seal between the face and the mask using the thumb and index fingers to form a "C" on the top of the mask, applying downward pressure while simultaneously using the middle, third, and fourth fingers under the mandible to pull it up to form a seal.[17] The right hand then squeezes the bag to deliver a breath. If using the two-person technique, one person creates the "C" on both sides of the face mask using both hands while using both hands to pull the mandible forward as described.[16,17] The adequacy of BVM is assessed by watching the rise and fall of the chest as would be done for mouth-to-mask ventilation. If the chest is not rising with ventilation, reposition the head and reattempt ventilation; if not successful (and there is no foreign body obstruction), an adjunct airway, such as an oropharyngeal (oral airway) or nasopharyngeal airway (nasal airway), may be required.[16,17]

Oropharyngeal and nasopharyngeal airways are adjuncts that assist in maintaining an unobstructed airway. Oropharyngeal airways should only be used for an unconscious patient because in partially responsive patients with intact airway reflexes, the oral airway can cause gagging, vomiting, and possibly laryngospasm, a condition whereby the vocal cords close and prevent ventilation.[16]

Oropharyngeal airways are available in multiple sizes, but the most commonly used adult sizes are 80, 90, 100 mm. To properly size the oral airway, place the flange of the airway at the corner of the patient's mouth. The curved end should reach the angle of the mandible.[15,16] The proper techniques for insertion are to use a tongue blade to hold the tongue down and forward while inserting the airway or by turning the airway upside down (curve facing up) toward the hard palate during insertion into the oral cavity and then rotating 180° once past the posterior portion of the tongue for proper placement in the posterior pharynx.[15,16] An improperly sized oral airway, either too large or too small, may cause trauma to the tissues and/or obstruct the airway by pushing the base of the tongue posteriorly.[16]

The nasopharyngeal airway, also called the nasal trumpet, is more pliable and can be tolerated by awake or semiconscious patients.[18] Common adult sizes are 6, 7, and 8 cm. Select the proper size by aligning the flange of the nasal trumpet with the exterior nare; the curved tip should reach the tip of the ear.[15,16] Attention should be given to the diameter of the nasopharyngeal airway, as it should be slightly smaller than the patient's nares; as the internal diameter increases, so does the length of the nasal trumpet.[16] Water-soluble lubricant should be applied to the nasal airway before insertion.[15] Using a gentle motion, insert through the nostril in a perpendicular plane in relation to the face following the floor of the nasopharynx. If resistance is encountered, you may try rotating the airway or attempting the other nostril.[16] Although the nasopharyngeal airway is usually well tolerated, it can still cause vomiting or laryngospasm.[16] The use of a nasopharyngeal airway should be avoided in anyone with facial fractures, as it may enter the cranial vault if basilar skull fracture is present.[15] Additional contraindications include patients who are anticoagulated or those patients with coagulopathic disease, as bleeding may occur.[18] Most important is to call for help if a patient is deteriorating, which entails contacting the physician for further orders and/or, if rapid deterioration of respiratory status is imminent, activating the rapid response team.

Preparation for intubation

If the patient requires intubation of the airway, it is essential that the RN be familiar with equipment, medications, and how they can best prepare for an emergent intubation procedure. Many rapid response teams will arrive with needed equipment and adjunct medication; nonetheless, the RN should collect an array of airways, endotracheal tubes, and stylets for the endotracheal tube. It is important to have this equipment available should the team arrive without equipment, or if difficulty is encountered, additional equipment is available. Adequate continuous suction should be available at the patient's head.[19] Be sure to check that the batteries/light is functional on the laryngoscope handle and blade. **Table 4** provides a guide to the equipment needed for intubation of the trachea.[19]

Medications

If the patient is conscious, medications may be necessary to secure the patient's airway. Medications to secure the patient's airway are more comfortable for the

Table 4 Equipment for tracheal intubation	
Airway Equipment	**Ancillary Equipment**
Endotracheal tubes sizes: 6.5, 7.0, 7.5, 8.0 mm	Oxygen source and nut and stem oxygen adapter
Laryngoscope blades: Macintosh 3 and 4; Miller 2 and 3. Laryngoscope handle	Yankauer suction tip, suction source and tubing, flexible suction tip
Oral and nasal airways	Carbon dioxide detector; waveform capnometry or colorimetric carbon dioxide device
10-cc syringe	Stethoscope
Stylets	
Ambu bag	
Ventilator	

patient but additionally may be safer and less traumatic. The most commonly used types of drugs used to secure the airway are sedatives, induction agents, and muscle relaxants.[19,20] The medications chosen depend on the patient's medical condition as well as the health care provider's knowledge and experience with various types of medications. Propofol is a drug used as an induction agent to render patients unconscious for general anesthesia but can also be used in reduced doses to provide sedation.[19,20] Propofol is a frequent choice for providing sedation or an unconscious state. This medication can cause severe hypotension; therefore, blood pressure monitoring and drugs to treat hypotension should be readily available.[19,20] Etomidate is another induction agent that is selected because it provides the patient with more cardiovascular stability than propofol.[19,20] A benzodiazepine, such as midazolam in lower doses, can provide adequate anxiety relief and amnesia for the patient during airway manipulation without producing unconsciousness or apnea.[19,20]

Muscle relaxants may also be used to relax the muscles of the airway and provide optimal intubating conditions.[19,20] Succinylcholine is a depolarizing muscle relaxant, and rocuronium is a nondepolarizing muscle relaxant.[19,20] Both medications provide muscle relaxation (paralysis) but through different mechanisms of action. Succinylcholine is not reversible but provides excellent intubating conditions within 60 seconds, and its duration of action is only 4 to 6 minutes.[19,20] However, this medication can cause bradycardia, has several contraindications, and carries a black box warning for the pediatric population.[19,20] Rocuronium is a nondepolarizing muscle relaxant with fewer adverse reactions and contraindications than succinylcholine but generally has a slower onset of action and a longer duration of action.[19,20]

It should be noted that these medications should only be administered by qualified health care personnel that are able to adeptly manage and secure the airway. Nurses should be aware of the effects these medications have on the patient: sedation, unconsciousness, and paralysis.

SUMMARY

Professional nurses, because of the continuous care they provide for patients, are pivotal in recognizing both subtle and major changes in the condition of their patients. Thus, it is necessary for nurses to recognize the signs of respiratory distress, to know how to physically assess their patients, and to be well versed in laboratory studies that can indicate impending respiratory deterioration. These skills will equip the nurse to act proactively to prevent further deterioration or arrest of the patient. A knowledge of various oxygen delivery systems can assist the nurse in understanding the relationship between Fio_2 and oxygen delivery in order to optimize the condition of the patient. The ability to properly manage the airway through BMV could save a patient's life until the rapid response team arrives to continue lifesaving efforts. Furthermore, a knowledge of the essential equipment needed for advanced airway management can improve the efficiency with which a secure airway is achieved.

CLINICS CARE POINTS

- Early signs of respiratory distress are dyspnea, disorientation, and tachycardia.
- Later signs of respiratory failure include slow breathing rate and bradycardia.
- Various types of oxygen delivery include low flow, high flow, and reservoir.
- The highest Fio_2 provided by low flow nasal cannula is 44%.

- Two-person bag mask ventilation is the best technique to ensure adequate ventilation.
- Oropharyngeal airways should only be used for the unconscious patient.
- Nasopharyngeal airways can be used with caution in the conscious or semiconscious patient.
- Continuous suction at the head of the patient is critical to preparation for intubation of the trachea.

REFERENCES

1. Jungquist CR, Smith K, Nicely KL, et al. Monitoring hospitalized adult patients for opioid-induced sedation and respiratory depression. Am J Nurs 2017;117(3 Suppl 1):S27–35.
2. Vo P, Kharasch VS. Respiratory failure. Pediatr Rev 2014;35(11):476–84 [quiz: 485–6].
3. Singh Lamba T, Sharara RS, Leap J, et al. Management of respiratory failure. Crit Care Nurs Q 2016;39(2):94–109.
4. Flenady T, Dwyer T, Applegarth J. Accurate respiratory rates count: so should you! Australas Emerg Nurs J 2017;20(1):45–7.
5. Elliott M, Baird J. Pulse oximetry and the enduring neglect of respiratory rate assessment: a commentary on patient surveillance. Br J Nurs 2019;28(19): 1256–9.
6. Fleming S, Thompson M, Stevens R, et al. Normal ranges of heart rate and respiratory rate in children from birth to 18 years of age: a systematic review of observational studies. Lancet 2011;377(9770):1011–8.
7. Mattar I, Liaw SY, Chan MF. Nurses' self-confidence and attitudes in using the Glasgow Coma Scale: a primary study. Nurs Crit Care 2015;20(2):98–107.
8. Gaines K. Know your ABGs - arterial blood gases explained. 2020. Available at: Nurse.org; https://nurse.org/articles/arterial-blood-gas-test/. Accessed December 22, 2020.
9. Kaufman D. Interpretation of arterial blood gases (ABGs). 2020. Available at: Thoracic.org; https://www.thoracic.org/professionals/clinical-resources/critical-care/clinical-education/abgs.php. Accessed December 22, 2020.
10. Miller K. Oxygen administration: what is the best choice? RT Web site. 2015. Available at: https://rtmagazine.com/products-treatment/monitoring-treatment/therapy-devices/oxygen-administration-best-choice/. Accessed November 25, 2020.
11. Fuentes S. Fraction of inspired oxygen. In: Chowdhury YS, editor. StatPearls [Internet]. Treasure Island (FL): StatPearls Publishing; 2020.
12. Hardavella G, Karampinis I, Frille A, et al. Oxygen devices and delivery systems. Breathe (Sheff) 2019;15(3):e108–16.
13. Blakeman TC, Branson RD. Oxygen supplies in disaster management. Respir Care 2013;58(1):173–83.
14. Spoletini G, Alotaibi M, Blasi F, et al. Heated humidified high-flow nasal oxygen in adults: mechanisms of action and clinical implications. Chest 2015;148(1): 253–61.
15. Barker S. Intermediate life support for the adult. Br J Nurs 2019;28(4):226–8.
16. American Heart Association. Management of respiratory arrest. Advanced cardiac life support; provider manual. Dallas (TX): First American Heart Association Printing; 2016. p. 47–55.

17. Meissen H, Johnson L. Managing the airway in acute care patients. Nurse Pract 2018;43(7):23–9.
18. Bullard D, Brothers K, Davis C, et al. Contraindications to nasopharyngeal airway insertion. Nursing 2012;42(10):66–7.
19. Dalley KB, Tola DH, Kesten KS. Providing safe passage: rapid sequence intubation for advanced practice nursing. AACN Adv Crit Care 2012;23(3):270–83.
20. Groth CM, Acquisto NM, Khadem T. Current practices and safety of medication use during rapid sequence intubation. J Crit Care 2018;45:65–70.

A Review of Best Practices Related to Intravenous Line Management for Nurses

Robingale Panepinto, DNP, FNP*, Jill Harris, MSN, RN,
Jessica Wellette, DNP, APRN, WHNP-BC

KEYWORDS

- Vascular access • Peripheral and central catheters/lines • PIV and CVC guidelines
- Protocols • PIV and CVC infection • Education • Training

KEY POINTS

- Specialized education for health care providers in peripheral intravascular (PIV) and central intravenous (CVC) catheter use, procedures, maintenance, and infection control.
- Utilize a specialized team for insertion and maintenance of CVCs and provide nurse training and checkoffs in PIV care.
- Nurses have an obligation to use evidence-based standards when inserting and maintaining peripheral and central venous lines.
- Proper insertion site choice is vital to patient safety as related to catheter function and avoidance of catheter-related infections.

INTRODUCTION

In the United States, at least 200 million peripheral intravascular (PIV) catheters are placed each year,[1] and it is estimated that more than 5 million central intravenous (CVC) catheters are placed annually.[2] It is also important to note that 60% to 90% of hospitalized patients will require a PIV catheter at some point in their treatment.[3] Intravenous access lines are an essential component of patient care and are used for administering parenteral medications, fluids, nutrition, and blood products. However, intravenous lines are not limited to hospitalized patients. They are also used in a variety of patient care settings, including outpatient infusion clinics, diagnostic radiology, urgent care facilities, and in-home care settings. Multiple types of intravenous access devices are available for use, and the choice of which type to use is determined by factors such as reason for placement, vasculature, and anticipated length and type of therapy. Short-term fluid infusions or medications in an acute care setting

Vanderbilt University School of Nursing, 461 21st Avenue South, Nashville, TN 37240, USA
* Corresponding author.
E-mail address: robingale.panepinto@vanderbilt.edu

Nurs Clin N Am 56 (2021) 389–399
https://doi.org/10.1016/j.cnur.2021.05.001
0029-6465/21/© 2021 Elsevier Inc. All rights reserved.

are often delivered via PIV catheters, whereas longer treatment regimens requiring vasopressors or irritant solutions may require CVCs.

HISTORY

The Infusion Nurses Society (INS)[4] publishes evidence-based best practice standards concerning all aspects of intravenous therapy and updates them approximately every 5 years. The authors used the most recently published Infusion Therapy Standards of Practice[4] as the starting point for their inquiry about best practices for nurses regarding management of intravenous access lines. The Centers for Disease Control and Prevention (CDC)[5] also published guidelines regarding safe and effective intravenous line management that the authors also referenced as they identified best practices. In 2012, the Joint Commission on Accreditation of Healthcare Organizations published a monograph entitled, "Preventing Central Line-Associated Bloodstream Infections: A Global Challenge, A Global Perspective," which was also reviewed. In addition, the authors conducted searches within the Cochrane Library, UpToDate, CINAHL, PubMed, and Medline databases. They used a variety of terms related to intravenous safety, complications, procedures, and maintenance to identify recent research and guidelines regarding best practices related to the prevention of complications associated with the use of peripheral and central venous lines.

DEFINITIONS
CLABSI

Central line–associated bloodstream infection: a primary bloodstream infection in a patient who had a central catheter within the 48-hour period before the development of the bloodstream infection and is not related to an infection at another site.

PIV

Peripheral intravenous catheter: a short catheter that is inserted into a vein of the peripheral circulation for the purpose of delivering fluids, medications, or solutions directly into the circulation.

CVC

Central venous catheter: an intravenous access device that terminates in the central circulation, typically in the superior vena cava. There are multiple types of central venous catheters, including surgically implanted catheters, tunneled catheters, nontunneled catheters, and peripherally associated central catheters.

PICC

Peripherally inserted central catheter: a long flexible catheter that is most often inserted in the basilic, cephalic, median cubital, or brachial vein and terminates in the superior vena cava or the junction of the superior vena cava and right atrium. PICC lines are a form of central venous access, and they are inserted using full surgical asepsis and maximal barrier methods.

Nontunneled CVC

A central venous catheter that is typically inserted into the subclavian, internal jugular, or femoral vein and ends in the central circulation. CVCs may terminate in the superior vena cava, in the junction of the superior vena cava and right atrium, or in the right atrium itself. Nontunneled CVCs are inserted using full surgical asepsis and maximal barrier methods.

BACKGROUND

Despite their widespread use, intravenous lines are not without risks and are a potential source for infection and complications. One study found that PIV failure rates and complications were as high as 53% in hospitalized patients.[6] Another study found that up to 69% of patients experience complications with their PIV, including but not limited to infiltration, extravasation, blockage, dislodgement, and phlebitis.[7] Data[8] also found that infection rates are as high as 5% to 25% at the time of removal. Patients with PIV-associated complications have longer hospital stays, have higher inpatient costs, and are at a greater risk of mortality than patients without such complications.[2] Unfortunately, this can delay procedures or drug administration and pose potentially significant burdens to health care personnel and systems.[9]

Although all types of vascular access catheters are associated with potential risk for localized infection or catheter-related bloodstream infections, CVCs carry a higher risk for bloodstream infections than PIVs, as they reside in large vessels within the central circulatory system. A single CLABSI can add 7 to 20 days to a hospital stay,[3] with costs[10] averaging $46,000. According to the Agency for Healthcare Research and Quality,[11] a branch of the United States Department of Health and Human Services, CLABSIs result annually in 84,551 to 203,916 preventable infections, 10,426 to 25,145 preventable deaths, and 1.7 to 21.4 billion dollars in avoidable costs to the United States. With this information in mind, nurses have an obligation to uphold evidenced-based standards to decrease the risk of infection and complications associated with intravenous lines. Infection risks and complications can be decreased by staying current in the evidence and ensuring evidenced-based standards are used within their own facility.

DISCUSSION
Peripheral Intravenous Catheters

Site selection and insertion
When PIV placement is required, the nurse must assess the patient's vasculature, health history, and reasons for placement. The appropriate gauge catheter will depend on what fluids or medications will be infusing through the vein and the patient's overall health status.[4] There are many factors and recommendations to take into consideration when deciding where to place a PIV. The INS states that health care professionals should "use the venous site most likely to last the full length of the prescribed therapy."[4] The INS also recommends inserting PIVs in the forearm, as they are generally more stable, have longer dwell times. and do not interfere as much with activities of daily living.[4] Their guidelines[4] also suggest consideration of the "dorsal and ventral surfaces of the upper extremities, including the metacarpal, cephalic, basilic, and median veins" and do not endorse the use of veins in the lower extremities for adult patients.

The CDC recommends[5] using the "upper extremity," whereas other research[12] recommends placement of PIVs in upper extremities, beginning with the distal veins and moving proximally. Both the INS[4] (2016) and UpToDate[12] (2020) suggest that joints or areas of flexion should be avoided, as catheters in these sites are prone to movement, occlusion, and dislodgement. When evaluating the patient for an insertion site, using landmark techniques can also help ensure the most appropriate vein is selected. This means that when looking for a vein, consider and assess the patient's overall health status, age, skin variations and alterations, body habitus, fluid status, and signs of previous drug use.[4] Previous puncture sites, scars, and tattoos should also be avoided.[4] Once a PIV site has been selected, no more than 2 attempts should be made by a single nurse and no more than 4 attempts in total.[4] Multiple attempts at PIV access can be painful to the patient, delay treatment, and increase costs.[4]

Skin asepsis

Variances in practices related to PIV placement are common, even among nurses that work on the same unit. However, as in Foley catheter placement, nurses should be knowledgeable of evidenced-based standards when inserting PIVs and ensure those standards are being implemented within their facility. Infection control measures and aseptic technique are essential when placing PIVs to prevent infection at the insertion site. Nurses must perform hand hygiene using either soap and water or an alcohol-based hand rub, and clean gloves should be donned before PIV insertion.[4,5] Excessive hair should be clipped to decrease the risk of accidently cutting the skin and serving as an open source for infection.[4]

For skin asepsis, the CDC recommends[5] using 70% alcohol, tincture of iodine, iodophor, or chlorhexidine gluconate to clean the skin before PIV insertion. However, the INS recommends[4] a solution of greater than 5% chlorhexidine in alcohol. Once the site has been cleaned, the site should not be palpated again before insertion to prevent infection.[4,5] When preparing the skin for a PIV, the circular motion has long been used by nurses. The rationale is that repeating this circular motion over the insertion site is effective in removing bacteria from the top layer of skin. There has been some evidence published on this technique in the past, but the authors were unable to find any current literature (published within the last 5 years) that supports this method. The CDC guidelines do not provide details on how to clean the insertion site; however, the INS recommends[4] a back-and-forth scrubbing technique. This technique is more effective at removing bacteria than a circular motion because it disinfects up to the first 5 dermal layers of the skin.[13] Data[13] noted that there was only 1 study that specifically compared these 2 cleaning techniques. This study compared culture contamination rates in an emergency department and found a statistically significant decrease from 3.5% to 2.2% when using a back-and-forth motion with chlorhexidine as compared with a circular motion[14] using tincture of iodine. Further research comparing these 2 cleaning techniques using chlorhexidine and alcohol would help strengthen evidence-based standards surrounding infection control for PIV insertion.

Dressings and stabilization

Adequate catheter dressing and securement are essential for maintaining[15] catheter integrity and reducing complications. When applied and maintained correctly, PIV site dressings and securement devices improve longevity, reduce the risk of dislodgement, and prevent[3] bacteria from contaminating the insertion site. Nonsterile tape is not recommended; however, engineered stabilization devices (ESDs) can be used in addition to PIV site dressings to promote[4] stabilization of the catheter. Catheter stabilization prevents[5] irritation of the vessel, dislodgement, or kinking of the catheter. The research[4] also recommends 1 of 2 options for PIV catheter stabilization: a peripheral catheter hub combined with a bordered polyurethane securement dressing or a standard round hub peripheral catheter in combination with an adhesive ESD. Tightly rolled bandages to secure[4] the PIV should not be used because it can limit visualization of the site and obstruct circulation. If the dressing becomes wet, loosened, or visibly soiled, the dressing should be changed.[4] Last, the dressing should always be dated[4] based on site-specific organizational policies.

Assessment

Nursing assessment of a PIV's dressing and securement is an integral component of promoting patient safety. INS guidelines[4] state that PIV catheters should be assessed at least every 4 hours, and more frequently based on the patient status and hospital guidelines. Assessment should involve visual inspection and palpation of the insertion site for redness, swelling, drainage, or tenderness. When continuous fluids are not infusing, function of the PIV should be assessed[5] before each use by aspirating and flushing the catheter. Finally, the CDC[5] encourages nurses to include their patient in teaching signs and symptoms of infection, or infiltration and dislodgement.

Dwell time/removal

The CDC[5] supports replacement of PIVs no more frequently than 72 to 96 hours. Researchers[4,5] agree that PIVs should not be replaced unless clinically warranted. Furthermore, the guidelines[4] state that PIV catheters should be removed when no longer necessary for a patient's plan of care or when clinically indicated based on "site assessment and/or clinical signs and symptoms of systemic complications."

Table 1 provides a summary of evidence-based practice recommendations for peripheral intravenous catheters in accordance with the INS, CDC, and UpToDate. The table addresses peripheral intravenous catheter site, skin preparation, dressing and securement, and removal or replacement.

Table 1
Summary of evidence based practice/recommendations: peripheral intravenous catheters

	Infusion Nurses Society	Centers for Disease Control and Prevention	UpToDate
Site	Forearm; dorsal and ventral surfaces of upper extremities AVOID: ventral surface of wrist, areas of flexion	Upper extremity	Distal veins in upper extremity should be used first; dorsal metacarpal, cephalic, median antebrachial (forearm)
Skin preparation	>0.5% chlorhexidine in alcohol solution; allow to dry	70% alcohol, tincture of iodine, or alcohol + chlorhexidine gluconate solution	>0.5% chlorhexidine preparation with alcohol
Dressing	Not specified	Sterile gauze or sterile, transparent, semipermeable dressing	Sterile gauze or sterile, transparent, semipermeable dressing
Dressing change	Change when soiled or loose, or at least every 5–7 d	Replace catheter site dressing if the dressing becomes damp, loosened, or visibly soiled	Do not remove/ change unless damp, loose, or visibly soiled
Securement	Engineered stabilization device or medical adhesive + transparent occlusive dressing	Sterile gauze or sterile, transparent, semipermeable dressing to cover the catheter site	Tape, prefabricated adhesive dressings, or specific intravenous securing devices
Removal or replacement	Remove/replace when clinically indicated (malfunction, complication)	Replace every 72–96 h (replacement based on clinical indication is identified as an "unresolved issue")	Remove/replace when clinically indicated

Peripheral intravascular bundles to reduce infection

The CDC recommends[5] the utilization of bundle strategies for PIV insertion within health care settings to encourage compliance with best practices. Hospitals from various countries have implemented[16] these care bundles into their practice and were collectively noted in a systematic review. There were some variances[16] among the studies used in the systematic review; however, some commonalities included use of 2% chlorhexidine gluconate, hand hygiene, site selection strategies, and utilization of closed catheters and transparent film dressings. The chart compares 2 of the studies conducted on adults in the United States that were evaluated in the systematic review.

Table 2 provides a summary of peripheral intravenous bundles according to study and author, setting, population, bundle components, findings, and conclusion.

Table 2
Examples of peripheral intravascular bundles

Study	A bundled approach to decrease the rate of primary bloodstream infections related to peripheral intravenous catheters	Protected clinical indication of peripheral intravenous lines: successful implementation
Authors	Duncan et al,[17] 2018	DeVries et al, [18] 2016
Setting	A nonprofit tertiary care trauma 1 center in a large metropolitan area of the Midwest with >9000 patient beds	A community hospital with >625 beds located in Northwest Indiana
Population	The 7-mo period resulted in 1977 peripheral and 378 central lines audits	Specific population size not mentioned, methods discussed
Bundle components	• Assess PIV sites and remove intravenous catheters if there is an indication of phlebitis • Ensure the dressing is dry, occlusive, and intact and change the dressing if it is nonocclusive or blood is present • Use alcohol-impregnated disinfecting caps on all needleless connectors • Minimize intravenous tubing disconnections • Use alcohol-impregnated disinfecting tip protectors on all disconnected intravenous tubing	• Staff education • Chlorhexidine gluconate skin preparation • Sterile gloves • Intravenous catheter with integrated extension set • Chlorhexidine gluconate–impregnated sponge dressing • Securement dressing • Alcohol disinfection caps
Findings	• 81% reduction in peripheral line–associated bloodstream infections compared with the preintervention period (from 0.57 to 0.11 infections per 1000 patient-days; $P<.001$) • 6% increase in the number of PIVs without pain, redness, or swelling (92% preintervention to 98% postintervention)	• 37% ($P = .03$) reduction from 0.052 out of 100 patient-days to 0.033 out of 100 patient-days in central and peripheral line infections • 19% reduction from 0.0150 out of 100 patient-days to 0.0121 out of 100 patient-days specifically in PIVs

Central Venous Catheters

Site selection and insertion

CVC insertion[19] often uses teams with specialized training in surgical asepsis. Maximum sterile barrier precautions, including the use of a body drape, mask, gown, cap, and sterile gloves, should be adhered to for insertion and dressing changes for all CVCs. Ultrasound guidance[19] is frequently used to avoid numerous insertion attempts and to decrease the risk of infection or complications in CVC placement. Although nurses are not typically responsible for the insertion site selection for CVCs, it is imperative that they are aware of how this indwelling line can cause infection. Some risks related to CVC site selection include infection, artery puncture, vein laceration, thrombosis, and catheter misplacement. To avoid contamination, CVCs should be inserted[19] as far from open wounds and burns as possible. For nontunneled CVC placement,[5] the CDC recommends the subclavian site over the jugular and femoral veins. Although the right basilic vein is considered,[20] this is the vein of choice for PICC placement because of its larger size and superficial location. Interestingly, a US hospital survey[21] found that 60% of hospitals use PICC teams for placement of central catheters.

Skin asepsis

According to the CDC guidelines,[5] aseptic technique is essential before accessing a CVC and before line replacing, repairing, or redressing at the site. According to researchers,[4,5] the skin should be prepared with greater than 0.5% chlorhexidine preparation with alcohol and allowed to dry before CVC placement. In the case of contraindications[5] to chlorhexidine, tincture of iodine, iodophor, or 70% alcohol may be used. Research[22] has shown a reduction in CLABSI rates for hospitalized patients with CVCs when general body skin is cleansed daily with a 2% chlorhexidine gluconate solution. The guidelines[5] also recommend the same for daily skin cleansing to reduce the incidence of CLABSIs. Daily bathing with a chlorhexidine gluconate solution[22] or skin care with chlorhexidine gluconate–impregnated bath wipes has become a standard of care for patients with CVCs in many facilities.

Dressings and stabilization

Catheter securement devices[19] are recommended to prevent migration, dislodgement, and factors that contribute to catheter malfunction, infiltration, and CLABSIs. Sterile dressings are used to cover CVC sites and are changed[5] according to the type used and the condition of the dressing. If transparent dressings are used, guidelines[4,5,23] all recommend chlorhexidine-impregnated dressings or the use of chlorhexidine sponges at the insertion site. These sources also state that in addition to changing the dressings whenever soiled or loose, gauze dressings should be changed every 2 days, and transparent occlusive dressings should be changed every 5 to 7 days using a sterile technique.

Assessment

For CLABSI prevention, CVC insertion sites[19] should be clean, dry, intact, and assessed for signs and symptoms of infection or migration daily. Staff training and education on line maintenance and protocols further assure the CLABSI prevention protocols are being adhered to. Patient education is also essential for patient safety and infection control. CVCs should be removed[5] as soon as they are no longer necessary for the patient's medical plan of care.

Dwell time/removal

Dwell time for CVCs are determined[5] based on continued need and assessment findings that indicate infection or complication. According to research,[23] the risk of CVC-related infection increases with the duration of use, but there are no standard recommendations regarding timelines or routine replacement. Careful assessment[5] and consideration of infectious and possible noninfectious sources should be ruled out before removal of a CVC. Because CVCs pose a higher risk for infection, frequent and daily assessment is recommended as a standard of care. CVCs should be removed[5] as soon as they are no longer necessary for the patient's medical plan of care.

Table 3 provides a summary of evidence-based practice recommendations for central venous catheters in accordance with the INS, CDC, and UpToDate. The table addresses central venous catheter site, skin preparation, dressing and securement, and removal or replacement.

Fig. 1 represents a mapping summary of best practice technique for peripheral intravenous catheters and central venous catheters.

FUTURE DIRECTIONS

There have been numerous studies evaluating the effectiveness of chlorhexidine compared with alcohol and betadine for central line placements. However, few studies specifically focus on how these findings relate to PIV placement. More research specifically focusing on this would be useful and supportive to strengthen guidelines and evidenced-based standards surrounding PIVs. One such research study that is

Table 3
Summary of recommendations: central venous catheters

	Infusion Nurses Society	Centers for Disease Control and Prevention	UpToDate
Site	Nontunneled CVC: Subclavian vein PICC: Median cubital, cephalic, basilic, or brachial vein	Subclavian vein	Non-tunneled CVC: Subclavian or internal jugular vein PICC
Skin preparation	>0.5% chlorhexidine in alcohol solution	>0.5% chlorhexidine in alcohol solution	Chlorhexidine (>0.5% CHG + alcohol)
Dressing type	Chlorhexidine-impregnated dressing Sterile gauze dressing if drainage is present	Chlorhexidine-impregnated dressing	Sterile gauze dressing, sterile CHG impregnated dressing, or CHG sponge at insertion site
Dressing change	Transparent: every 5–7 d Gauze: every 2 d AND/OR when soiled or loosened	Transparent: every 7 d Gauze: every 2 d AND/OR when soiled or loosened	Transparent: every 7 d Gauze: every 2 d AND/OR when soiled or loosened
Securement	Adhesive engineered stabilization device	Sutureless securement device	Not indicated
Removal or replacement	Assess justification for CVC daily; remove when no longer needed for plan of care	Not indicated	Remove as soon as clinically feasible

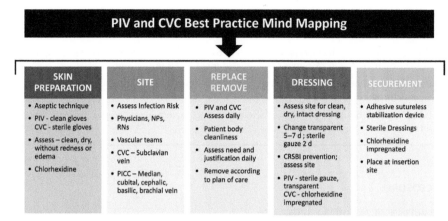

Fig. 1. Mapping summary for peripheral intravenous catheter and central venous catheter best practice technique. CRSBI, catheter related blood stream infection; NPs, nurse practitioners; RNs, registered.

specifically focusing on antisepsis for PIV placement is the CLEAN 3 Protocol Study that started in April 2019. The preliminary article reported that the study[24] will be composed of 1000 patients from a hospital emergency room and is an open-label, single-center, randomized, 2-by-2 factorial trial. This study[24] will specifically evaluate the antisepsis rates between 2% chlorhexidine-alcohol and 5% povidone iodine–alcohol for skin preparation for PIVs. Results of this study have not yet been published; however, findings[24] from this research study will further contribute to the evidence behind infection control for PIV placement.

CURRENT EVIDENCE

A common theme throughout published literature is the recommendation for the establishment and consistent use of specialized teams of health care professionals trained in placement and maintenance of intravenous lines. Evidence shows a specialized vascular access team contributes to the reduction in CLABSIs. Patient safety, complications, and health care costs directly relate to the adherence to protocols,[19] training, education, checklists, and maintenance of PIV and CVC lines.

SUMMARY

Vascular access device complications and best practice is a topic commonly discussed and well documented throughout medical and nursing literature. The placement, utilization, and maintenance of both peripheral and central access devices all pose potential patient health risks. Nurses have an obligation to provide safe patient care and adhere to the most current evidence-based standards when caring for patients with intravenous lines. Using resources such as the INS and CDC for education and training of nurses in the areas of PIV and CVC insertion, technique, assessment, and maintenance is imperative to reduce infection rates of patients in the health care setting.

CLINICS CARE POINTS

- Ensure evidence-based standards are being adhered to within health care facilities to maintain and decrease the risk of infection with intravenous lines.

- Chlorhexidine is recommended for site preparation and maintenance of peripheral intravascular and central intravenous catheters.
- The back-and-forth technique is preferred over the circular technique for peripheral intravascular/central intravenous catheter skin asepsis at insertion sites.
- Possible intravenous complications include infiltration, extravasation, dislodgement, and venous thrombosis.
- Hand hygiene should be performed before inserting, maintaining, or accessing intravenous lines.

DISCLOSURE

The authors have nothing to disclose.

REFERENCES

1. Patel S, Alebich M, Feldman L. Routine replacement of peripheral intravenous catheters. J Hosp Med 2017;12:42–5.
2. Lim S, Gangoli G, Adams E, et al. Increased clinical and economic burden associated with peripheral intravenous catheter-related complications: analysis of a US hospital discharge database. Inquiry 2019;56:1–14.
3. Helm RE, Klausner JD, Klemperer JD, et al. Accepted but unacceptable: peripheral IV catheter failure. J Infusion Nurs 2019;42(3):151–64.
4. Infusion Nurses Society. Infusion therapy standards of practice 2016. Available at: https://source.yiboshi.com/20170417/1492425631944540325.pdf.
5. Centers for Disease Control. Guidelines for the prevention of intravascular catheter-related infections 2017. Available at: https://www.cdc.gov/infectioncontrol/pdf/guidelines/bsi-guidelines-H.pdf.
6. Steere L, Ficara C, Davis M, et al. Reaching one peripheral intravenous catheter (PIVC) per patient visit with LEAN multi-modal strategy: the PIV5Rights™ bundle. J Assoc Vasc Access 2019;24(3):31–43.
7. Marsh N, Webster J, Larson E, et al. Observational study of peripheral intravenous catheter outcomes in adult hospitalized patients: a multivariable analysis of peripheral intravenous catheter failure. J Hosp Med 2018;13(2):83–9.
8. Zingg W, Pittet D. Peripheral venous catheters: an under-evaluated problem. Int J Antimicrob Agents 2009;34(4):S38–42.
9. Morrell E. Reducing risks and improving vascular access outcomes. J Infusion Nurs 2020;43(4):222–8.
10. Haddadin Y, Annamaraju P, Regunath H. Central line associated blood stream infections. StatPearls; 2020. Available at: https://www-ncbi-nlm-nih-gov.proxy.library.vanderbilt.edu/books/NBK430891/.
11. Agency for Healthcare Research and Quality. Appendix 2. Central line-associated bloodstream infections fact sheet 2018. Available at: https://www.ahrq.gov/hai/clabsi-tools/appendix-2.html.
12. Frank R. Peripheral venous access in adults. UptoDate; 2020. Available at: https://www.uptodate.com/contents/peripheral-venous-access-in-adults?search=peripheral%20venous%20access&source=search_result&selectedTitle=1~150&usage_type=default&display_rank=1#H27755089.
13. Stonecypher K. Going around in circles: is this the best practice for preparing the skin? Crit Care Nurs Q 2009;32:94–8.

14. Tepus D, Fleming E, Cox S. Effectiveness of Chloraprep in reduction of blood culture contamination rates in emergency department. J Nurs Care Qual 2008;23(3): 272–6.
15. Corley A, Ullman AJ, Mihala G, et al. Peripheral intravenous catheter dressing and securement practice is associated with site complications and suboptimal dressing integrity: a secondary analysis of 40,637 catheters. Int J Nurs Stud 2019;100:1–10.
16. Ray-Baruel G, Xu H, Marsh N, et al. Effectiveness of insertion and maintenance bundles in preventing peripheral intravenous catheter-related complication and bloodstream infection in hospital patients. A systematic review. Infect Dis Health 2019;24(3):152–68.
17. Duncan M, Warden P, Bernatchez SF, et al. A bundled approach to decrease the rate of primary bloodstream infections related to peripheral intravenous catheters. J Assoc Vasc Access 2018;23(1):15–22.
18. DeVries M, Valentine M, Mancos P. Protected clinical indication of peripheral intravenous lines: successful implementation. J Assoc Vasc Access 2016;21(2): 89–92.
19. O'Grady NP, Alexander M, Burns LA, et al. Summary of recommendations: guidelines for the prevention of intravascular catheter-related infections. Clin Infect Dis 2011;52(9):1087–99.
20. Gonzalez R, Cassaro S. Percutaneous central catheter. StatPearls; 2020. Available at: https://www.ncbi.nlm.nih.gov/books/NBK459338/.
21. Krein SL, Kuhn L, Ratz D, et al. Use of designated nurse PICC teams and CLABSI prevention practices among U.S. hospitals: a survey-based study. J Patient Saf 2019;15(4):293–5.
22. Dombecki C, Sweeney J, White J, et al. CHG skin application in non-ICU patients with central venous catheters: impact on CLABSI, MRSA bacteremia, and LabID Rates. Infect Control Hosp Epidemiol 2020;41(S1):S164–5.
23. Jacob JT, Gaynes R. Intravascular catheter-related infection: prevention. UptoDate; 2019. Available at: https://www.uptodate.com/contents/intravascular-catheter-related-infection-prevention?search=intravascular%20catheter-related%20infection:%20Prevention&source=search_result&selectedTitle=1~150&usage_type=default&display_rank=1.
24. Guenezan J, Drugeon B, O'Neill RO, et al. Skin antisepsis with chlorhexidine-alcohol versus povidone iodine-alcohol, combined or not with use of a bundle of new devices, for prevention of short-term peripheral venous catheter-related infectious complications and catheter failure: an open-label, single-centre, randomised, four-parallel group, two-by-two factorial trial: CLEAN 3 protocol study. BMJ 2019;9(4):1–8.

Educational Theory and Cognitive Science
Practical Principles to Improve Patient Education

Margaret (Betsy) Babb Kennedy, PhD, RN, CNE*,
Abby Luck Parish, DNP, AGPCNP-BC, GNP-BC, FNAP

KEYWORDS

• Cognitive science • Patient education • Adult learning • Learning styles

KEY POINTS

- Provision of effective patient education is a hallmark of quality care that can significantly impact patient satisfaction and outcomes.
- Nurses can plan for more effective patient teaching and improved learning outcomes using adult learning and cognitive science principles.
- Knowledge of cognitive load theory can inform design of patient learning experiences to facilitate learning goals.

INTRODUCTION

Nurses play a trusted and critical role in educating patients and their families to support improved health outcomes. Every nurse is expected to plan, implement, and evaluate strategies for patient learning, often under challenging conditions. In the 10 years since the article Assessing Patient Learning Styles: Practical Tips for Patient Education[1] was published, there is now greater understanding of both cognitive science and the importance of empowering patients as central to health-care decision-making through patient-centered education. Further, advances in technology have created multiple media opportunities to enhance educational approaches. The purpose of this article is to extend the practical tips of the previous article with an introduction to educational theory and cognitive science principles for consideration in improving the effectiveness of patient education.

BACKGROUND

Provision of effective patient education is a hallmark of quality care that can significantly impact patient satisfaction and outcomes. In the previous article, the reader

Vanderbilt University School of Nursing, 274 SON, 461 21st Avenue South, Nashville, TN 37240, USA
* Corresponding author.
E-mail address: Betsy.kennedy@vanderbilt.edu

Nurs Clin N Am 56 (2021) 401–412
https://doi.org/10.1016/j.cnur.2021.04.006
0029-6465/21/© 2021 Elsevier Inc. All rights reserved.

was introduced to adult learning principles, as well as motivation and readiness for learning.[1] Adult learners are motivated to learn for the purpose of changing their knowledge, skills, or behavior related to a specific and important need to do so.[2,3] In the health-care setting, adult patients would be motivated to learn as the result of a need to manage their own health and participate fully in health-care decisions.[4] Their orientation for learning is goal driven, with the need for specific knowledge and skills that will be immediately applicable. Readiness is also a concept applied to adult learning and closely linked to the need to know.[2–4] It is conceivable that although one may be motivated to learn, they may not be ready, with barriers commonly being related to health issues. Adult learners also value autonomy in learning, making decisions about what, how, and when it takes place.[2–4] However, many times, in the patient education context, there is no ability to set these parameters, creating obstacles to learning.[5]

The previous article also introduced the reader to assessment factors for consideration in planning patient education, including biophysical, psychological, social, cultural, and environmental domains.[1] Over the past decade, the necessity and value of this holistic assessment has been affirmed by the movement in health care toward patient-centered care. An essential first step in patient-centered education is assessment of patient learning needs using principles of cultural humility, which is defined as the intent to listen to and honor patients' beliefs, customs, and values.[6] Trauma-informed care principles may be integrated for patients who disclose or have a known history of trauma.[7] Patient communication and education have been proposed as strategies to reduce health inequities, but in order for education to effectively address disparities, nurses must begin with listening and holistic assessment.[8,9]

Nurses can plan for more effective patient teaching and improved learning outcomes by remembering principles of adult learning and grounding strategies in educational theories and cognitive science principles. What follows is a review of concepts and theories from the science of learning that are foundational to adult education.

CONSTRUCTIVISM

Constructivism is a theory consistent with adult learning principles about how individuals learn by actively constructing their own understanding based on previous experiences, knowledge, and preconceptions.[10–12] New information from teaching is then connected and reconciled with what the learner already knows.[13] If the learner's fundamental conceptions are sound and correct, new knowledge and understanding can then be built on this foundation. Misconceptions can prevent assimilation of new information if learners believe the new information to be false, erroneous, or otherwise incompatible with their previous understanding.[12,13] Therefore, faulty misconceptions can impact the effectiveness of the teaching and impact patient outcomes.

Nurses can use a constructivist approach in an educational encounter by asking what previous experiences the patient has had or knowledge that might be relevant to the situation. In dialog with the patient, existing knowledge can be used to frame activities and new information, and gaps in knowledge and misconceptions can be identified and addressed as needed. When misconceptions are present and new information conflicts with previous knowledge, cognitive dissonance can result.[14] The patient must then choose to accept the new information or reject it in favor of their previous beliefs, rendering teaching ineffective. Using questioning that elicits rationale, that is, why questions, the nurse can help patients generate answers themselves, which will support acceptance of the new information through teaching.

For example, an obstetric nurse is working with an interdisciplinary team to discuss the implications of preterm delivery for a fetus at 26 weeks of gestation. The patient's sister delivered a premature infant at 27 weeks of gestation 5 years earlier, and that child has, to her knowledge, no long-term complications. Although the length of time in the neonatal intensive care unit was difficult for the family, the patient does not have any other experience or knowledge of prematurity and makes an assumption that her pregnancy ending early will have a similarly positive outcome. The team is presenting new information that challenges the beliefs of the patient and her family, resulting in cognitive dissonance. Asking probing questions about the previous experience and rationale for beliefs can help reset the patient's foundation for learning.

ACTIVE LEARNING

Constructivist approaches are generally linked to active learning strategies. Active learning strategies can be described as those that support the learner in constructing knowledge rather than a simple transmission of knowledge.[15] Activities can vary, but all are designed to prompt the learner to connect previous and new knowledge. Examples include pausing to ask for reflection or quick recall on what was just taught and the inclusion of case scenarios. The social and cooperative aspect of learning is also part of active learning with group/peer teaching strategies to support learning outcomes.[16]

Frequently, patient education involves verbal instruction from the nurse to the patient and family in a format similar to a short lecture, with printed materials available to support the teaching. Unless active strategies are used, this amounts to transmission of knowledge that results in less retention of knowledge.[17] Nurses can easily include brief pauses during patient teaching to ask for recall or return demonstration of a skill. When teaching, the nurse can incorporate different scenarios related to possible complications or troubleshooting equipment/devices and ask the patient about appropriate steps to take to problem-solving.

For example, a nurse providing family education about communicating with a loved one with dementia could begin by providing information about using warm facial expressions and body language while meeting the person with dementia in whatever reality they are experiencing without the need to reorient them. The nurse can then ask the family members to describe a situation in which communicating with the person with dementia was frustrating or difficult. The nurse can then ask the family members for ideas for navigating a similar situation in the future by incorporating the principles that they have learned. This discussion personalizes the education to the family's unique challenges and engages them in actively troubleshooting for future interactions.

LEARNING STYLES AND LEARNING PREFERENCES

Learning styles have been broadly described as patterns of learner preferences for instruction. There are numerous learning style models and frameworks that attempt to characterize how learners organize and store information for future use. In the previous article, the VARK framework by Fleming and Mills[18] is presented as a popular and accessible way to identify learner preferences and inform teaching approaches.[1] To review, VARK represents sensory modalities of learning: Visual, Auditory, Reading (or Writing), and Kinesthetic. Those who identify as visual learners prefer information depicted in pictures such as charts or symbols. Auditory learners have a preference for processing information through hearing the spoken word such as discussion. Some learners prefer information processing through reading written text as is the form of much of patient education materials. Finally, kinesthetic learners prefer a tactile and physical processing of information with practice. However, most individuals can be multimodal with strengths across modes and not limited to any one mode.

Learning styles have been the subject of debate in education. There is a noted lack of evidence for improved learning outcomes when teaching to a particular known learning style preference.[19] Thus, teaching to a preferred style rather than based on best strategies for the particular information that needs to be taught is not ideal. Patients may not be aware of a particular learning style preference or have a particular learning skill set for different learning capabilities. It is important to remember that if patients state they have a preferred learning style, it does not mean that adapting teaching to that style will result in any different learning outcomes. However, knowing the patient's preferred learning style may help to include teaching activities or materials to which the patient will be more receptive. Learning preferences can be considered helpful in balancing design approaches to patient teaching, but not essential to improving patient outcomes. The primary objective is for the educator to design teaching and learning strategies effective for the topic and context rather than for the learner to focus on learning through a primary preferred style.

METACOGNITION

Metacognition is the act of thinking about one's own thinking. It is a cognitive process that includes awareness of one's self as a learner. More specifically, it involves the ability to identify gaps in understanding and learning needs, setting goals for learning, engaging in learning activities, and monitoring progress toward achieving learning goals.[20] It is a dynamic and ongoing process that involves learners understanding their strengths and weaknesses as a learner.[21] While this process is learner centered, the nurse can engage patients in conversation that promotes thinking about how they learn best, how they identify gaps in learning, and how they will know that they have been successful in learning. Certain activities of learning can promote metacognition. As previously discussed, asking the patient what they already know about the relevant topic encourages reflection on past learning. Periodically asking the patient during teaching what is still unclear can help with identifying gaps. Asking patients to summarize their learning and how their thinking may have changed after the teaching encounter also encourages reflection on what was learned and how.

Desirable difficulties

The concept of desirable difficulties refers to the challenges and frustrations imposed in the process of learning new information or skills, and that engagement with some difficulty can promote deeper learning.[22] While learners generally enjoy the easiest path to learning, more challenging tactics that promote encoding and retrieval of information can be more beneficial.[23] Active learning practices such as the following examples support desirable difficulties. However, the challenges imposed by the circumstances requiring patient education must be balanced with imposing additional challenges on the learning encounter.

Retrieval Practice

Retrieval practice is a study strategy for learners that involves trying to recall information without having it present in order to promote long-term retention.[24,25] Retrieval practice is essentially repeatedly testing oneself on information to remember facts. When used in the classroom, retrieval-based learning can be seen as frequent quizzing or practice testing. Learners can also use retrieval practice in the form of self-quizzing that can help identify knowledge gaps for future study. In the context of patient education, when the goal is long-term retention of important information such as self-management of diabetes in education after initial diagnoses, the nurse can design teaching sessions that allow for asking questions that prompt patient retrieval of facts. Retrieval practice may be enhanced by stating the learning objectives for the teaching session prior to starting to help guide the patient learner's attention.

Teach-back is frequently used to determine patients' understanding or comprehension of education by asking them to restate or summarize what has been taught back to the educator.[26,27] This type of retrieval practice is demonstrated to be effective with patients of all ages and health literacies.[28,29] Without a retrieval practice such as teach-back, patients' first attempt at recall may be at the time that they need the information. Prompting retrieval of the information immediately after the patient receives it allows initial retrieval to occur in a low-stakes setting and promotes longer retention of education.

Spaced Learning

Spaced learning is a strategy whereby the learner studies material or practices a skill in spaced intervals of time rather than in one single session to promote long-term retention of information.[25,30] Even short intervals between learning sessions can have great impact. For example, patient education that included three 5- or 10-min sessions spaced apart would yield better knowledge retention than one 15- or 30-min session.

Deliberate Practice

Practice and repetition of a skill is essential to mastery, and deliberate practice is practice with the intention of improvement in a systematic and purposeful way. Deliberate practice is also linked to motivation and challenging oneself despite associated difficulties. Deliberate practice has been linked to learner qualities of grit and growth mindset.[31] Grit is the quality of pursuing goals with dedication,[32] and growth mindset is the notion that intelligence is malleable rather than fixed.[33] Guiding learners to engage in deliberate practice for difficult tasks prompts them to engage fully and take risks and in doing so affirms a growth mindset and encourages grit.[34]

COGNITION

A summary for each of the identified theories or concepts from cognitive science is provided, along with tips for application and examples of use in patient education.

Cognitive Load Theory

Cognitive load theory asserts that there are multiple components to memory (**Fig. 1**). Sensory memory is the component that is responsible for collecting information through auditory or visual channels. It is transient, with some information selected for input to working memory. Working memory temporarily stores and processes information from sensory input and integrates it with information retrieved from long-term memory about what is already known in real time. New understanding is then encoded and returned to long-term memory. Although the capacity of long-term memory is practically limitless, the capacity of the working memory is finite.[35] Therefore, when considering the experience of learning and the limits of processing in working memory, the concept of cognitive load becomes critical. During instruction, the demands on working memory are called the cognitive load.[36–39] If the cognitive load is too high, learning cannot occur; however, the components can be

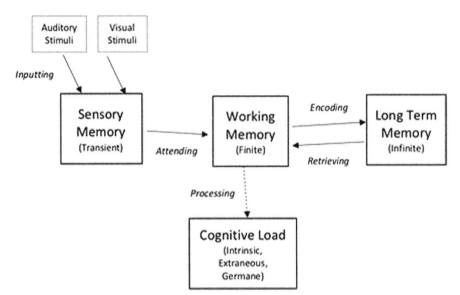

Fig. 1. Cognition. (*Adapted From* Brame, CJ. Effective educational videos. 2015. Retrieved January 1, 2021 from http://cft.vanderbilt.edu/guides-sub-pages/effective-educational-videos/.)

manipulated though intentional design of patient education experiences to support learning.[40,41]

The three components of cognitive load include the intrinsic load, extraneous load, and germane load and are described in **Table 1**. The intrinsic load is the difficulty of the learning task or the subject itself (Sweller 1994; Sweller 1998). For example, consider the difference between basic math (1 + 1 = 2) and inferential statistics or learning the signs and symptoms of infection (redness, drainage, fever) for a postoperative incision and a family member caregiver managing jejunostomy tube feedings. Intrinsic load is generally fixed.[38,39] Therefore, design of a teaching plan or material would need to address the other components of cognitive load to facilitate meaningful learning.

Extraneous load refers to information that requires cognitive processing effort but does not contribute to the learning objective.[40] Nonessential details, confusing instructions, and environmental factors such as timing, noise, stress, or privacy issues can all distract the learner and interrupt processing. Germane load is the cognitive processing required to meet the objective, constructing schema through analysis of ideas and recognizing connections for learning.[36] It can be manipulated by breaking down a

| Table 1 |
| Components of cognitive load |

Component	Description	Nature
Intrinsic Load	Inherent difficulty of the learning task	Nonmodifiable
Extraneous Load	The manner in which the information is presented to the learner	Modifiable
Germane Load	The level of information processing activity necessary for learning	Modifiable

complex learning task into smaller, more manageable tasks to support overall learning and integration.

With knowledge of cognitive load theory, the nurse can consider the limitations of working memory, the level of difficulty of the task/information, and the context or setting for teaching and make decisions about the learning experience design to facilitate encoding to long-term memory and enhance learning.

For example, a patient's partner tells the nurse that they have just learned the patient has a terminal diagnosis and that they have questions about the end-of-life trajectory and exactly how much time the patient might have left. The nurse knows that the intrinsic load of end-of-life changes and prognosticating is high. The nurse also recognizes that the partner's extraneous load is very high owing to having received bad news. Taking into account germane load, the nurse begins by allowing partners to express their feelings and then teaches the partner a simple beginning strategy for assessing patient changes as a measure of remaining life (ie, that persons experiencing declining changes month to month often have months to live, persons experiencing declining changes week to week often have weeks to live, and so forth). The nurse plans to return frequently to provide support and more education as the partner processes the extraneous load of the news.

Dual Code Theory

Aligned with cognitive load theory, dual code theory suggests that working memory has two distinct and independent cognitive channels for information processing: the text/audio channel and the visual channel.[42] Incoming auditory information is placed on a sequential loop.[42] Concurrently, incoming visual information such as words or images is committed to a visual sketchpad, with a symbolic picture in working memory that can potentiate the auditory imagery.[42,43] The two independent sources of information are linked for encoding and transfer to the long-term memory, with two distinct pathways for later, more efficient, retrieval.[42] If there is congruency between the auditory and visual information, learning is maximized.[44,45] Conversely, if there is incongruence in the visual and auditory information, meaningful connection is impeded.[44] Thus, although working memory remains limited in capacity, when the capacities of both sensory input channels are used effectively together in parallel, information uptake can be enhanced.[44]

Multimedia Learning Theory

Building on both cognitive load theory and dual code theory, the cognitive theory of multimedia learning states that there is an optimal and appropriate combination of visual and auditory mediums that can enhance learning.[45,46] Frequently, multiple materials and multimedia methods are used for patient education. Together, the three theories presented offer useful information for maximizing effectiveness of patient teaching and learning. Supportive strategies are summarized in **Table 2**.

For example, the nurse creates a brief video designed for persons initiating treatment with selective serotonin reuptake inhibitors. To reduce extraneous load, the video includes animations demonstrating pathophysiology and video of persons experiencing treatment and adverse effects, while a voice provides description so that the learner has congruent but nonduplicative visual and auditory input. To further reduce extraneous load, the video does not include background music and is only 4 minutes long. To address germane load, the video begins with basic pathophysiology principles and builds to an explanation of desired treatment responses. To address intrinsic load, the nurse provides brief education including key principles during a brief face-to-face encounter, followed by providing the patient with a link (on

Table 2	
Educational strategies to address cognitive load components	
Cognitive Principle	Supportive Educational Strategies
Extraneous Load	• Use both text and graphics simultaneously to augment learning by giving patients the written/visual materials at the same time as verbal instruction. • Ensure text and verbal (or narration) instruction are congruent, but not redundant. • Place the corresponding text and graphics closer together rather than far apart. • Eliminate music and other background on recorded presentations. • Reduce distractors in the setting for learning. • Highlight key points.
Germane Load	• Highlight key words and elements for emphasis on organization and relationships.
Intrinsic Load	• Provide definitions of key words ahead of teaching. • Organize teaching in segments. • Offer patients some control regarding pace of the teaching encounter and flow of information. • Deconstruct complex tasks/information into smaller chunks. • Allow patients to have some control over timing of teaching and amount of information.

printed materials and via email through the patient portal). Patients are encouraged to view the video when time allows or when patients have questions, and they are also advised to directly contact the nurse with follow-up questions or needs.

DISCUSSION

Multiple contexts and circumstances can influence the design of patient education with adult learners. Time, timing, and health literacy are noted barriers to effective patient education.[47–50] A collaborative and individualized approach that includes assessment of previous knowledge, appropriate spacing, and reinforcement of teaching, with feedback and evaluation after teaching at appropriate intervals, does not occur quickly or haphazardly. Ideally, discharge planning and patient teaching begins on admission. In the event of known procedures or events, education about care issues that will affect health outcomes can be initiated proactively with multiple opportunities for teaching. When various factors limit time, effective teaching and learning outcomes can still be achieved. It is most important to view effective patient education not as a single encounter but rather as a longitudinal process.[49]

The key to designing effective patient education is to focus on the learning objective. Learning objectives can be related to communication of information for decision-making in the short term or mastery of skills or procedures that will be essential for long-term care. The context of timing, time available, complexity of the content or skills, as well as the multiple patient variables must all factor in the design and implementation of patient education.

The foundation of patient education is clear communication, and most patient education, at least initially, is verbal.[51] Education may be implemented in person or, with the advent of telehealth, virtually. In either setting, use of an approachable,

conversational tone during the interaction is preferable. Clarity of text in patient education materials, whether print or across multiple modalities, is also critical in consideration of cognitive load.[52] Additional concerns related to communication include health literacy language, culture, and physiologic barriers.[47] Thorough assessment of multiple dimensions that can influence patient education can support an individualized, culturally sensitive, understandable approach to teaching strategies to meet the learning objective.[1]

Demonstration of skills, graphic print materials, and videos and other multimedia methods, even simulation[53] and virtual reality,[54] can be used in effective patient and family education in a multidisciplinary approach.[49] However, when multiple modalities are used for patient education, they must be explained as to purpose and instructional use. Effective patient education is dependent on alignment of clear learning objectives, evidence-based teaching strategies, and appropriate educational resources.[55]

Multiple modalities should also be assessed for accessibility considerations and adjusted to meet individual patient needs. Accessibility is generally understood as the degree to which services or materials can be used by all intended audiences (https://accessiblecampus.ca/understanding-accessibility/). In education, barriers to accessibility are usually related to the sending or receiving of information that can impact communication. Examples of accessible patient education materials include the provision of resources such as documents that can be interpreted by screen readers for visually impaired patients, closed captioning or video transcripts for hearing impaired patients, and self-paced modules for persons with limited energy or attention.

SUMMARY

Safety and quality improvement initiatives to improve patient-centered health-care delivery frequently include elements of patient education as central to patient satisfaction and outcomes. Effective patient education should inform and empower patients in meeting specific objectives for optimizing health care. Effective education begins with holistic and patient-centered assessment of prior experiences and learning needs. Using principles of constructivism, nurses can build on those previous experiences and support patients to integrate new knowledge and skills. Active learning engages learners to be independent problem-solvers after discharge. While in the past, patient education may have been geared to learning preferences, nurses have the opportunity to instead prioritize principles of cognitive science in order to deliver education that takes into account variables such as extraneous, intrinsic, and germane load. Grounding patient education approaches in practical, yet evidence-based and science-backed, strategies can improve effectiveness and health-care outcomes.

CLINICS CARE POINTS

- Use of active learning strategies can help patients build new knowledge and promote long term retention.
- Nurses should consider the limits of working memory, the difficulty of the task/information, and the context for teaching when planning patient learning experiences.
- Patient learning outcomes can be optimized using a patient centered approach, clear objectives, and consideration of cognitive science principles.

DISCLOSURE

The authors have nothing to disclose.

REFERENCES

1. Inott T, Kennedy B. Assessing learning styles: practical tips for patient education. Nurs Clin North Am 2011;46:313–20.
2. Knowles MS. Modern practice of adult education: from pedagogy to andragogy. 2nd edition. New York: Cambridge Books; 1980.
3. Knowles MS, Holton EF, Swanson RA. The adult learner: the definitive classic in adult education and human resourced development. 7th edition. Burlington (MA): Elsevier, Inc; 2011.
4. Twaddell JW. Educating parents about vitamin K in the newborn using Knowles' theory of adult learning principles as a framework. Crit Care Nurs Q 2019;42(2): 205–7.
5. Lasa-Blandon M, Stasi K, Hehir A, et al. Patient education issues and strategies associated with immunotherapy. Semin Oncol Nurs 2019;35(5):150933.
6. Stubbe DE. Practicing cultural competence and cultural humility in the care of diverse patients. Focus (Am Psychiatr Publ) 2020;18(1):49–51.
7. Ranjbar N, Erb M, Mohammad O, et al. Trauma-informed care and cultural humility in the mental health care of people from minoritized communities. Focus (Am Psychiatr Publ) 2020;18(1):8–15.
8. Ogbogu PU, Capers Q, Apter AJ. Disparities in asthma and allergy care: what can we do? J Allergy Clin Immunol Pract 2020;9(2):663–9.
9. Jain J, Moroz L. Strategies to reduce disparities in maternal morbidity and mortality: patient and provider education. Semin Perinatol 2017;41(5):323–8.
10. Brandon AF, All AC. Constructivism theory analysis and application to curricula. Nurs Educ Perspect 2010;31(2):89–92.
11. Weidman J, Baker K. The cognitive science of learning: concepts and strategies for the educator and learner. Anesth Analg 2015;121(6):1586–99.
12. Dennick R. Constructivism: reflections on twenty five years teaching the constructivist approach in medical education. Int J Med Educ 2016;7:200–5.
13. Nowicka-Sauer K, Jarmoszewicz K, Trzeciak B, et al. Constructivism in patient education: using drawings to explore preconception of coronary artery disease. Kardiol Pol 2018;76(8):1274–6.
14. Festinger LA. Theory of cognitive dissonance. Stanford (CA): Stanford University Press; 1957.
15. Ambrose SA, Bridges MW, DiPietro M, et al. How learning works: seven research-based principles for smart teaching. San Francisco (CA): Jossey-Bass; 2010.
16. Tsiamparlis-Wildeboer AHC, Feijen-De Jong EI, Scheele F. Factors influencing patient education in shared medical appointments: integrative literature review. Patient Educ Couns 2020;103(9):1667–76.
17. Fritschi C, Martyn-Nementh P, Zhu B, et al. Active learning: lessons from women with type 2 diabetes in a walking program. Diabetes Educ 2019;45(4):370–9.
18. Fleming ND, Mills C. Not another inventory, rather a catalyst for reflection. To Improve the Academy 1992;11(1):137–55.
19. Pashler H, McDaniel M, Rohrer D, et al. Learning styles: concepts and evidence: concepts and evidence. Psychol Sci Public Interest 2008;9(3):105–19.
20. Bransford J, Brown A, Cocking R. How people learn: Brain, mind, experience, and school. Washington, DC: National Academy Press; 2000.

21. Pintrich PR. The role of metacognitive knowledge in learning, teaching, and assessing. Theory Into Practice 2002;41(4):219–25.
22. Bjork EL, Bjork RA. Making things hard on yourself, but in a good way: creating desirable diffculties to enhance learning. In: Gernsbacher M, Pomerantz J, editors. Psychology and the real world: essays illustrating fundamental contributions to society. New York: Worth; 2014. p. 56–64.
23. Steenhof N, Woods NN, Mylopoulos M. Exploring why we learn from productive failure: insights from the cognitive and learning sciences. Adv Health Sci Educ Theory Pract 2020;25(5):1099–106.
24. Roediger HL 3rd, Karpicke JD. The power of testing memory: basic research and implications for educational practice. Perspect Psychol Sci 2006;1(3):181–210.
25. Roediger HL III, Pyc MA. Inexpensive techniques to improve education: applying cognitive psychology to enhance educational practice. J Appl Res Mem Cogn 2012;1:242–8.
26. Shersher V, Haines TP, Sturgiss L, et al. Definitions and use of the teach-back method in healthcare consultations with patients: a systematic review and thematic synthesis. Patient Educ Couns 2021;104(1):118–29.
27. Tamura-Lis W. Teach-Back for quality education and patient safety. Urol Nurs 2013;33(6):267–71, 298.
28. Centrella-Nigro AM, Alexander C. Using the teach-back method in patient education to improve patient satisfaction. J Contin Educ Nurs 2017;48(1):47–52.
29. Caplin M, Saunders T. Utilizing teach-back to reinforce patient education: a step-by-step approach. Orthop Nurs 2015;34(6):365–8.
30. Cepeda NJ, Pashler H, Vul E, et al. Distributed practice in verbal recall tasks: a review and quantitative synthesis. Psychol Bull 2006;132(3):354–80.
31. Park D, Tsukayama E, Yu A, et al. The development of grit and growth mindset during adolescence. J Exp Child Psychol 2020;198(104889):104889.
32. Duckworth AL, Peterson C, Matthews MD, et al. Grit: perseverance and passion for long-term goals. J Pers Soc Psychol 2007;92(6):1087–101.
33. Dweck C. Mindset: the new psychology of success. New York: Ballantine Books; 2008.
34. McClendon C, Grand Canyon University, Massey Neugebauer R, et al. Grit, growth mindset, and deliberate practice in online learning. Journal of Instructional Research 2017;6(1):8–17.
35. Baddeley A. Working memory. Science 1992;255(5044):556–9.
36. van Merriënboer JJG, Sweller J. Cognitive load theory in health professional education: design principles and strategies. Med Educ 2010;44(1):85–93.
37. Sweller J. Cognitive load during problem solving: effects on learning. Cognitive Science 1988;12(2):257–85.
38. Sweller J, van Merrienboer JJG, Paas FGWC. Cognitive architecture and instructional design. Educ Psychol Rev 1998;10(3):251–96.
39. Sweller J. Cognitive load theory, learning difficulty, and instructional design. Learning and Instruction 1994;4(4):295–312.
40. Chandler P, Sweller J. Cognitive load theory and the format of instruction. Cognit Instruct 1991;8(4):293–332.
41. Pusic MV, Ching K, Yin HS, et al. Seven practical principles for improving patient education: evidence-based ideas form cognition science. Paediatr Child Health 2014;19(3):119–22.
42. Paivio A. Dual coding theory: retrospect and current status. Can J Psychol 1991;45:255–87.

43. Baddeley A. The episodic buffer: a new component of working memory? Trends Cogn Sci 2000;4(11):417–23.
44. Mayer RE. Applying the science of learning: evidence-based principles for the design of multimedia instruction. Cogn Instruction 2008;19:177–213.
45. Mayer RE. Multimedia learning. 2nd edition. New York: Cambridge University Press; 2012.
46. Mayer RE, Moreno R. Nine ways to reduce cognitive load in multimedia learning. Educ Psychol 2003;38:43–52.
47. Beagley L. Educating patients: understanding barriers, learning styles, and teaching techniques. J Perianesth Nurs 2011;26(5):331–7.
48. Shlobin NA, Clark JR, Hoffman SC, et al. Patient education in neurosurgery: part 1 of a systematic review. World Neurosurg 2020. https://doi.org/10.1016/j.wneu.2020.11.168.
49. Shlobin NA, Clark JR, Hoffman SC, et al. Patient education in neurosurgery: part 2 of a systematic review. World Neurosurg 2020. https://doi.org/10.1016/j.wneu.2020.11.169.
50. Skelton SL, Waterman AD, Davis LA, et al. Applying best practices to designing patient education for patients with end-stage renal disease pursuing kidney transplant. Prog Transplant 2015;25(1):77–84.
51. Marcus C. Strategies for improving the quality of verbal patient and family education: a review of the literature and creation of the EDUCATE model. Health Psychol Behav Med 2014;2(1):482–95.
52. Wilson EA, Wolf MS. Working memory and the design of health materials: a cognitive factors perspective. Patient Educ Couns 2009;74(3):318–22.
53. Lefèvre T, Gagnayre R, Gignon M. Patients with chronic conditions: simulate to educate? Adv Health Sci Educ Theory Pract 2017;22(5):1315–9.
54. Pandrangi VC, Gaston B, Appelbaum NP, et al. The application of virtual reality in patient education. Ann Vasc Surg 2019;59:184–9.
55. Baker D, DeWalt D, Schillinger D, et al. "Teach to Goal": theory and design principles of an intervention to improve heart failure self-management skills of patients with low health literacy. J Health Commun 2011;16(sup3):73–88.

Preventing Catheter-Associated Urinary Tract Infections with Incontinence Management Alternatives
PureWick and Condom Catheter

Kimberly Bagley, DNP, AGPCNP-BC, AGACNP-BC, CCRN[a,b,*],
Lindsey Severud, BSN, RN, CCRN[c]

KEYWORDS

- CAUTI prevention • Use of external urinary collection devices • Condom catheter
- PureWick

KEY POINTS

- Catheter-associated urinary tract infections (CAUTI) have high direct and indirect costs for hospitals and increase mortality by 3 times.
- Nurses at the bedside use Best Practices in CAUTI prevention to promote patient safety for patients with urinary incontinence.
- Nurses play a key role in determining if indwelling urinary catheters or external urinary collection devices are appropriate for the patient.

INTRODUCTION/HISTORY/DEFINITIONS/BACKGROUND

Health care-acquired infections (HAIs) incur considerable expense for health care facilities and patients alike. Recognizing the considerable costs associated with HAIs, health care systems across the nation both individually and within nationally organized efforts through the Agency for Healthcare Research and Quality (AHRQ), Centers for Medicare and Medicaid Services, and the Health Research and Educational Trust (HRET) have worked to reduce HAIs. The national study, On the CUSP: Stop Blood Stream Infections campaign, proved how effective national campaigns can be with a 41% reduction in central line–associated bloodstream infections.

Catheter-associated urinary tract infections (CAUTIs) occur when an indwelling urinary catheter (Bard, Benton, Dickinson, and Company, Four Oaks, NC, USA) becomes

[a] Critical Care Medicine, Duke Health, Duke Raleigh Hospital, ATTN: DRAH ICU, 3400 Wake Forest Road, Raleigh, NC 27609, USA; [b] Duke University School of Nursing, Durham, NC, USA; [c] Intensive Care Unit, Duke Raleigh Hospital, ATTN: DRAH ICU, 3400 Wake Forest Road, Raleigh, NC 27609, USA
* Corresponding author.
E-mail address: kimberly.bagley@duke.edu

Nurs Clin N Am 56 (2021) 413–425
https://doi.org/10.1016/j.cnur.2021.05.002
0029-6465/21/© 2021 Elsevier Inc. All rights reserved.
nursing.theclinics.com

colonized with bacteria. *Escherichia coli* and *Staphylococcus* are 2 primary organisms that cause urinary tract infections (UTIs) and are becoming more difficult to treat with the overuse of antibiotics.[1,2] **Box 1** lists most commonly reported pathogens that cause CAUTI.[3] When HRET led the AHRQ-funded On the CUSP: Stop CAUTI project using the infrastructure in place from the previous On the CUSP: Stop Blood Stream Infections project, only modest reductions were achieved in CAUTI. These improvements were greatest within intensive care units (ICU).[4]

Organized efforts within a health care facility or through national efforts may be beneficial, but they often fail to recognize the impact of individual nursing care. These efforts tend to have a greater focus on knowledge, and less on individual behaviors. Even though it is estimated by the Society of Healthcare Epidemiology of America that as much as 69% of CAUTI can be prevented by using evidence-based strategies, it is important to note that many of the evidence-based recommendations focus on recognition of appropriate use of indwelling catheters and hands-on care (ie, hand hygiene, proper aseptic technique, good peritoneal care).[5–7]

Prevention strategies have heavily focused on health care provider knowledge, using didactic content to inform providers on the risk and impact of CAUTI, and on the use of bundles that include appropriate indications for indwelling urinary catheters, maintenance, and removal.[8–13] With this focus on shaping knowledge and practice, there has been less emphasis on understanding the motivation and social and environmental factors that play a role in acquiring CAUTIs. Recognizing that nurse knowledge and skill is not the only barrier to effective CAUTI prevention is important. Factors such as ease of use, the feeling that physicians are dictating nursing practice, lack of understanding of the severity of CAUTI, and the benefit of CAUTI prevention for the patients all should be recognized and addressed.[14]

UTIs cost about $5 billion in both indirect and direct costs yearly, and CAUTIs specifically account for between 30% and 40% of all HAIs in the United States.[2] Although the estimated expense associated with CAUTIs is commonly $1000, factors such as patient population, inpatient setting of ICU or non-ICU, infection with antibiotic-resistant organisms or susceptible strains, and cost perspective (such as private insurance vs Medicare, hospital charity care, and so forth) all influence the costs and can result in

---

Box 1
Most common catheter-associated urinary tract infections pathogens, 2015 to 2017

Escherichia coli

Selected *Klebsiella* spp

Pseudomonas aeruginosa

Enterococcus faecalis

Proteus spp

Enterobacter spp

Other *Enterococcus* spp

Coagulase-negative staphylococci

Enterococcus faecium

Citrobacter spp

Staphylococcus aureus

(Weiner-Lastinger, 2020.)

increases not generally accounted for.[15] Increased costs associated with hospitalizations can result in lower patient satisfaction, as patients are asked to pay the brunt of the expense, which then has a direct impact on hospital reimbursement and reputation.

With an estimated 70% of CAUTIs considered preventable by following evidence-based strategies, the CMS lists CAUTIs as having payment implications for hospitals.[16] In addition to the financial burden incurred with CAUTI and the impact on hospital reimbursement, patients can suffer dire consequences. CAUTIs are associated with a threefold increase in morbidity and mortality.[17] An estimated thirteen thousand patient deaths are associated with UTIs annually.[18] Treatment of CAUTIs also contributes dramatically to antibiotic resistance, both for the patient and for society as a whole.[2] **Table 1** lists reported pathogens that tested nonsusceptible to antibiotic agents.[3]

Table 1
Pathogens associated with catheter-associated urinary tract infections that tested nonsusceptible to antibiotic agents, 2015-2017

Pathogens	Antibiotic Agents with Resistance
Staphylococcus aureus	OX/CEFOX/METH (MRSA)
Enterococcus faecalis	Vancomycin (VRE)
Selected *Klebsiella* spp	ESCs Carbapenems (CRE) MDR
Escherichia coli	ESCs Carbapenems (CRE) FQs MDR
Enterobacter spp	Cefepime Carbapenems (CRE) MDR-2
Pseudomonas aeruginosa	AMINOS ESCs-2 FQs-2 Carbapenems-2 PIP/PTAZ MDR-3
Acinetobacter spp	Carbapenems-2 MDR-4
(Weiner-Lastinger, 2020)	

Abbreviations: AMINOS, Aminoglycocides (ex. Amikacin, gentamicin, tobramycin); Carbapenems-2 (ex. Imipenem, meropenem, or doripenem); PIP/PTAZ, piperacillin and piperacillin/tazobactam; CRE, Carbapenem-resistant Enterobacteriaceae (ex. Imipenem, meropenem, doripenem, or ertipenem); ESCs, extended-spectrum cephalosporins (ex. cefepime, cefotaxime, ceftazidime, or ceftriaxone); ESCs-2, extended-spectrum cephalosporins (ex. cefepime or ceftazidime); FQs, Fluoroquinolones (ex. ciprofloxacin, levofloxacin, moxifloxacin); FQs-2, Fluoroquinolones (ex. ciprofloxacin or levofloxacin); MDR, Multi-drug resistant (non-susceptible to 1 drug in at least 3 of the following classes: ESCs, FQs, Aminoglycocides, Carbapenems, piperacillin/tazobactam); MDR-2, Multi-drug resistant (non-susceptible to 1 drug in at least 3 of the following classes: Cefepime, FQs, Aminoglycocides, Carbapenems, piperacillin/tazobactam); MDR-3, Multi-drug resistant (non-susceptible to 1 drug in at least 3 of the following classes: ESCs-2, FQs-2, Aminoglycocides, Carbapenems-2, piperacillin and piperacillin/tazobactam); MDR-4, Multi-drug resistant (non-susceptible to 1 drug in at least 3 of the following classes: ESCs-2, FQs-2, Aminoglycocides, Carbapenems-2, piperacillin and piperacillin/tazobactam, ampicillin/sulbactam); MRSA, Methicillin-resistant Staphylococcus aureus; OX/CEFOX/METH, Oxacillin/Cefoxatin/Methicillin; VRE, Vancomycin-resistant Enterococcus.

Given the financial and human costs associated with CAUTI, nursing best practices have shifted toward noninvasive urinary management strategies to prevent CAUTI. Multimodal interventions have been evaluated to assess effectiveness in CAUTI reduction.[19] When the use of urinary catheters is indicated, strategies to reduce CAUTI include avoiding the use of indwelling urinary catheters, adherence to aseptic technique when catheter placement is necessary, maintaining proper care of urinary catheters and peritoneal hygiene, and removing catheters once no longer needed.[20] Multimodal evidence-based interventions have been shown to decrease HAIs. However, the preventable HAIs do not actually diminish over time, highlighting the need for continued research and diligence with infection prevention practices in the acute care setting.[21] Nursing plays a vital role in adherence to infection prevention practices, in patient and staff education, in bundle implementation, and in staff accountability.

Nursing has taken on a greater role in infection prevention practices within the inpatient setting. Throughout inpatient units, nurses serve as unit champions for CAUTI prevention, conduct audits to verify indwelling urinary catheters are indicated and have appropriate orders, and evaluate the need for indwelling catheters during daily rounds with providers. Nurses also work alongside infection prevention and hospital providers to devise new methods to reduce indwelling urinary catheter use, such as development of a registered nurse (RN)-driven Foley Protocol that allows nurses to assess the need for a urinary catheter on a daily basis and then to remove the catheter if it is no longer deemed necessary. Working at the bedside, nurses are in the unique position to understand patient limitations with self-care and activities of daily living and can identify the presence of urinary incontinence and if mentation is a factor. Identification of urinary incontinence is the first step in understanding the patient's needs. Once urinary incontinence has been identified, causes can be explored to determine best management strategies.

Urinary incontinence is the unintentional loss of bladder control resulting in passing urine. There are 5 common types of urinary incontinence, which are detailed in **Box 2**. Although urinary incontinence is often associated with old age, it is not a normal part of aging and can be avoided or reversed with measures such as bladder training, lifestyle changes, pelvic floor muscle training (Kegel exercises), or medications. Common causes of urinary incontinence vary based on the setting (inpatient vs outpatient), underlying conditions, and medication use.[16] **Table 2** provides list of common causes of urinary incontinence.

Box 2
Common types of urinary incontinence

Stress incontinence: Involuntarily passing of urine when there is a sudden strain, such as coughing or sneezing

Urge incontinence: The bladder is unable to control the impulse to urinate

Overflow incontinence: Urine retention causes the bladder to become distended, which leads to the bladder not being able to contract strongly enough to create a urine stream, which results in dribbling

Functional incontinence: Urine leaks despite a normally functioning bladder and urethra and is related to cognitive or mobility factors

Mixed incontinence: Symptoms of stress and urge incontinence in the same patient

Table 2 Common causes of urinary incontinence	
Underlying Conditions	**Medications**
Delirium or confusion	Diuretics (furosemide/Lasix, bumetanide/Bumex, torsemide/Demadex)
Dehydration	Hypnotics (zolpidem/Ambien, butabarbital/Butisol, flurazepam/Dalmane)
Childbirth	Sedatives (lorazepam/Ativan, alprazolam/Xanax, chlordiazepoxide/Librium, clonazepam/Klonopin, diazepam/Valium)
Fecal impaction	Anticholinergics (diphenhydramine/Benadryl, doxylamine/Unisom, glycopyrrolate/Robinul, hydroxyzine/Atarax, ipratropium/Atrovent, oxybutynin/Ditropan, tiotropium/Spiriva, bupropion/Wellbutrin, dextromethorphan (found in Delsym 12 hr/Robitussin)
Restricted mobility	
Diabetic neuropathy	
Prostatic hyperplasia	
UTI	
Guillain-Barré syndrome	
Urethral stricture	

GUIDELINES

There are several resources available for nurses and health care professionals to assist with management strategies for urinary incontinence. The Centers for Disease Control and Prevention (CDC) offers comprehensive guidelines for urinary incontinence management with indwelling urinary catheters. **Table 3** provides a summary of these recommendations.[6] Several organizations, such as American Urological Association, the Society of Urodynamics, the European Association of Urology, the Canadian Urological Association, the International Consultation on Incontinence, and the National Institute for Health and Care Excellence, all have recommendations for conservative management of urinary incontinence as well as medication therapy. **Table 4** provides a summary of these recommendations.[22]

DISCUSSION

Once urinary incontinence is identified, it is then necessary to identify the underlying cause to assist with management strategies. Nurses are often able to easily identify when confusion or delirium is a factor. When working with confused patients, nurses can set a schedule to encourage bladder emptying to prevent urinary retention and the need for indwelling catheters. This approach can increase patient safety by reducing agitation and attempts to get out of bed in the hospital when the need to urinate is the driving factor. Because the risk of patients pulling out indwelling urinary catheters increases for agitated or confused patients, nurses are the first line in patient safety to avoid potential harm and the risk of infection associated with indwelling urinary catheters for confused patients. This form of urinary incontinence, called functional incontinence, can be seen in the inpatient setting with delirious, confused, or sedated patients. Nursing strategies to assist with incontinence management include bladder training, diet and drug modifications, adequate hydration, minimizing use of incontinence pads/briefs as trapped moisture and heat can lead to skin breakdown, and if needed, external urinary devices.[16]

Table 3
Summary of Centers for Disease Control and Prevention guidelines for urinary catheter use, management, and management of urinary incontinence

Appropriate catheter use	Insert indwelling urinary catheters only when there is an appropriate indication
	Examples of appropriate indications: Acute urinary retention, bladder outlet obstruction, need for accurate urinary output in critically ill patients, perioperative use, healing open sacral or perineal wounds incontinent patients, prolonged immobility, end-of-life care
Use proper insertion techniques	Hand hygiene before insertion, insertion by properly trained and competent individuals only, use the smallest bore tube possible, use of aseptic technique and sterile equipment, securement to assist with stabilization and prevention of urethral traction
Catheter management	Replace the urinary catheter if there is a break in aseptic technique, the tubing becomes disconnected, there is infection, the collection system becomes compromised, or there is leakage
	Monitor for and take steps to prevent the tubing or collection system from kinking
	Keep the urinary collection device below the level of the bladder at all times
	Do not place the collection bag on the floor
	Empty the collection device regularly to prevent overflow and backflow of urine
	Do not use antiseptics to clean the periurethral area while the catheter is in place

CAUTI Guidelines. Centers for Disease Control and Prevention. https://www.cdc.gov/infectioncontrol/guidelines/cauti/index.html. Published November 5, 2015. Accessed November 29, 2020.

Prevention strategies for CAUTI include making sure that indwelling urinary catheters are placed with appropriate indications, making sure that reminders or prompts are in place for catheter removal once it is no longer indicated,[23] and providing regular education on CAUTI and its impact for the patient to medical staff. In an effort to reduce CAUTI, some organizations have empowered nursing with nurse-driven protocols through which nurses can remove indwelling urinary catheters once they are no longer indicated. These efforts in combination with catheter care bundles recognize the importance of nursing and the bedside care provided to patients. In addition to a focus on appropriate use of indwelling urinary catheters, evidence-based strategies also emphasize hands-on care, such as hand hygiene and good peritoneal care.[5]

Implementing these measures can be challenging, as nurses perceive a change in practice and become resistant to changes because of a lack of education or understanding of the severity of CAUTI. When units have an established protocol for chlorhexidine gluconate (CHG) baths, it is important that adequate CHG baths are given instead of the CHG cloth not being applied to the skin long enough to have a cleaning effect.[9] Another barrier that can arise is when nurses ignore reminders to remove catheters once no longer indicated, often because of the convenience of a catheter.[17]

When an indwelling urinary catheter is not indicated and the patient has urinary incontinence, an external urinary collection device can be used. This device collects urine in tubing or a bag using gravity or into a container using suction. For male

Table 4	
Guideline-based recommendations for treatment of urinary incontinence	
Conservative Management	**Medication Therapy**
Scheduled voiding for bladder training	Use nonpharmacologic strategies first
Fluid restriction	Use behavioral modifications in combination with medication therapy
Smoking cessation	Antimuscarinics as first- or second-line treatment of urge urinary incontinence
Avoid or minimize caffeine	Similar efficacy seen between antimuscarinics
Pelvic floor muscle therapy	Use intermediate release for initial therapy, then change to extended release if ineffective
>5% weight reduction	Extended release has less occurrence of dry mouth and so is preferred
Treatment of constipation	8- to –12-wk trial of medications is recommended to be able to assess for efficacy
For light urinary incontinence, use of containment devices or disposable pads	If ineffective or adverse drug effects, may modify dosing or try another antimuscarinic
For moderate to severe urinary incontinence, disposable pads, external devices, or indwelling urinary catheters	Use caution in the elderly
Posterior tibial nerve stimulation for urge urinary incontinence	May use duloxetine in stress and mixed urinary incontinence
	Medication therapy should be used for temporary improvement in urinary incontinence
	As a second-line medication for stress urinary incontinence, mirabegron can be used
	Desmopressin can be used for short-term relief
Syan, 2016	

patients, common external urinary collection devices include the condom catheter (Conveen, Coloplast company, Humlebaek, Denmark) and a male penis pouching system (BioRelief.com, Hollywood, FL, USA). For female patients, the PureWick device (Benton, Dickinson, and Company, Four Oaks, NC, USA) is a common external urinary collection device that sits outside of the urethra, have an absorbent pad on the end that collects urine, and is attached to suction that draws the urine into a canister that can then be measured. External urinary collection devices are best used in cooperative patients who do not have urinary retention or bladder outlet obstruction.[24] It is important to note that these devices can be easily removed by patients, result in less accurate urinary output measurements, and lead to unidentified urinary retention. They may be considered in the setting of neurogenic bladder dysfunction and reflex urinary incontinence, or as short-term drainage in patients with altered mentation during acute or chronic illness.[24]

CONSIDERATIONS

When using PureWick, it is important to make sure there is sufficient airflow around the pad that is placed against the urethra. It should not be used in conjunction with a bedpan. If a patient has a bowel movement, the PureWick should be completely changed out, to include the drainage tubing and suction canister. This device is not recommended in combative patients, those with history of recent urogenital surgery, or those with frequent bowel incontinence without a fecal management system in place.

Contraindications for condom catheters are latex/adhesive allergies, preexisting skin irritation or open lesions on the glans or penile shaft, phimosis/paraphimosis, catheter-induced hypospadias, and if the patient is confused/agitated enough to cause trauma via incorrect removal methods.

Patients with urinary retention should not have an external urinary collection device. Urinary retention should be treated with indwelling urinary catheter and have input from Urology.

APPLICATION

When applying a condom catheter or a PureWick, proper application is important. **Table 5** provides key points of application.[16] Once a device has been appropriately applied, it can become necessary to troubleshoot. If a condom catheter frequently comes off, evaluate if the appropriate size has been chosen. Male patients who have a retracted penis will not keep a condom catheter in place effectively, making a male penis pouching system necessary (**Fig. 1**). For the PureWick system, if urine is not being collected in the canister, the first step is to double check that the system is plugged in,

Table 5	
Key points to correct application of the condom catheter and the PureWick	
Condom Catheter with External Urinary Drainage Bag	**PureWick Female External Urinary Collection Device**
Choose the correct size for the patient's penis (small, medium, or large)	Clean the peritoneum and vagina with soap and water
For a circumcised patient, first wash the penis with soap and water, then rinse, and then pat dry	Check skin integrity before PureWick application
For an uncircumcised patient, retract the foreskin gently to clean underneath it, then rinse but do not dry. The moisture acts as additional lubrication and assists with preventing friction. Once clean and rinsed, gently replace the foreskin	Spread the patient's labia and buttocks to place the PureWick between the labia, with the tip close to the rectum
Once the penis is clean, apply the skin protectant	Do not place the PureWick into vagina or rectum
Insert the glans through the opening of the condom catheter and position the strip 1 inch from the scrotum	Check the suction settings, targeting intermediate and not high settings
There should be about one-half inch between the condom end and the tip of the penis so that urine can drain out of the urinary meatus When unrolling the condom catheter downward, press the sheath against the penis to improve the adhesive bond Using the extension tubing, connect the condom catheter to the urinary drainage bag Avoid twists in the extension tubing that could obstruct urine flow Keep the urinary drainage bag off the floor	Avoid twists in the extension tubing

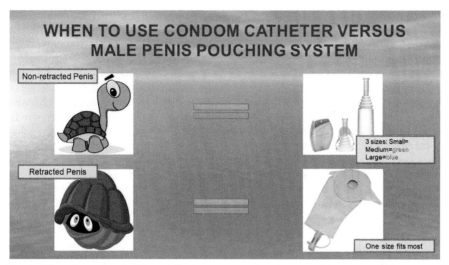

Fig. 1. When to use to condom catheter versus male urine pouching system. (*Courtesy of Amanda Elitz.*)

that the tubing is connected from the PureWick to the canister, and that the suction is turned on. If despite these steps no urine is being collected, it is important to evaluate the patient with a bladder scan to confirm the presence of urine or lack of, and to rule out urinary retention, which is a contraindication for external urinary collection devices.

COMPLICATIONS/CONCERNS

As with indwelling urinary catheters, there are potential complications with the use of external urinary collection devices. UTIs, skin breakdown, pressure injury, and localized trauma can all occur. Condom catheters can be challenging if the male anatomy hinders the ability to achieve an adequate seal on application. This can result in leaking and increase patient discomfort. Condom catheters can be used for 1 to 3 days, although they should be changed out and skin checks performed daily. External penis pouching systems can be used up to a week, but daily skin assessment is needed to prevent complications, such as skin breakdown and pressure injury. Use of the Pure-Wick device can result in skin breakdown if not changed regularly, and localized trauma to the tissue from the suction if settings are too high.

Regardless of the device, maintaining correct placement can be difficult when patients have altered mental status or other cognitive dysfunction. This can make it challenging to assess the patient's urine output and can result in complications, such as skin breakdown and localized trauma. Other complications, such as localized necrosis, gangrene, and yeast infection, have been found to occur as a result of urine leakage, poor hygiene, improper device application, and high suction settings. Nursing staff education on appropriate indications for external urinary collection devices, proper application and suction settings, peritoneal care, and skin checks is crucial to patient safety.

CASE STUDIES
Case Title: "Condom Catheter Pitfalls: Learning Opportunities"

Case presentation
A 78 year-old man with a past medical history of hypertension (HTN), hyperlipidemia (HLD), uncontrolled diabetes mellitus, and chronic obstructive pulmonary disease

(COPD) presented to the Emergency Department (ED) with hypoxia (SpO2 [peripheral capillary oxygen saturation] 70s) and respiratory distress. He was intubated in the ED and then transferred to the ICU for further management. While in the ICU, the patient remained intubated and sedated for 3 days, during which time a condom catheter was placed for urinary incontinence, and bladder scans were done every 6 hours to monitor for urinary retention. The patient's treatment course included intravenous (IV) steroids to treat COPD exacerbation and IV antibiotics. During the first 12 hours, the condom catheter came off and had to be replaced by the nurse. Thirty-six hours into his hospitalization, the condom catheter was pulled off by the patient as he started to wake up during a sedation wean. Forty-eight hours after admission, the patient was extubated. When the nurse worked with a colleague to give the patient a chlorhexidine bath, the condom catheter slid off. On inspection, the penis had 2 large skin tears weeping serous fluid, along with the skin over the head of the penis being red, which was concerning for skin breakdown.

Clinical questions

1. What complications occurred as a result of using a condom catheter?
2. What steps could have been taken to prevent these complications?
3. What other complications could arise from use of a condom catheter?

Discussion

This case highlights the potential for complications with condom catheter use for an intubated patient sedated in the ICU. Various potential complications with condom catheter use include skin tears, skin breakdown, and pressure injury. There is also a risk of increased skin breakdown or UTI with the penis head and urethra sitting in urine for extended periods of time if the catheter is not kept in a dependent position to allow for urine flow down the tubing into the drainage bag. Despite the risks involved with use of a condom catheter, with appropriate nursing care there still remains a significantly decreased chance of harm from use of a condom catheter in comparison to use of an indwelling urinary catheter. Choosing the correct size of the condom catheter in addition to appropriate use of adhesive during condom catheter placement, such as Mastisol, can minimize the likelihood of the condom catheter being removed by accident. During application of the condom catheter, it is possible for the foreskin to be pulled back, which can cause edema when the foreskin is not replaced. It is also possible for a pressure injury to occur on the underside of the penis from the condom catheter. Changing the condom catheter daily, with gentle removal to avoid skin tearing, allows for regular skin checks and minimizes infection risk. If there is concern for the patient pulling the condom catheter off, consideration should be given to use of an external urinary bag to avoid skin tears. For patients with a retracted penis, an external urinary bag is more appropriate than a condom catheter for management of urinary incontinence. Changing the bag and performing skin checks on a daily basis are equally as important when using an external urinary bag.

Case Title: "PureWick Pitfalls: Learning Opportunities"

Case presentation

A 64 year-old woman presented with a significant medical history of COPD, HTN, HLD, and recent history of a 30-day hospitalization during which time a PureWick was in place. She was discharged to a rehabilitation facility and then brought back to the hospital 2 days later with a UTI and fungal infection across the perineum and vagina.

Clinical questions

1. During the previous hospitalization, was the patient's PureWick changed at the appropriate frequency?
2. What complications occurred as a result of PureWick use?
3. What steps could have been taken to prevent these complications?

Discussion

Chart review of the previous hospitalization revealed that there was no documentation of the PureWick ever being changed by nursing, although it was documented that it was in use. It was unknown if the device had been changed and simply not documented, and so, if it had been changed, it was unknown if it had been done frequently enough. The patient was readmitted to the hospital with septic shock requiring vasopressors as a result of a UTI. She also required antifungal treatment for her fungal infection. Changing the PureWick device, tubing, and suction canister every 12 hours or as needed, such as with every bowel movement, along with regular skin checks could have potentially prevented these complications. Other considerations include the suction settings to ensure that the suction is not set too high, which can cause tissue damage, and that nursing care is appropriately documented.

This patient suffered a life-threatening complication from her PureWick use. Septic shock can result in patient death, even if appropriate antibiotics are started, fluid resuscitation is given, and vasopressors are used. The patient also had an increased risk of delirium from UTI and critical illness requiring care in the ICU. Changing the PureWick device, tubing, and suction along with skin checks could have prevented the complications resulting in hospitalization. It is important to note that the lack of appropriate nursing documentation makes this case difficult, as it is unknown if appropriate nursing care was provided. Accurate documentation is the only way to be able to determine if appropriate care has been received.

SUMMARY

Best practices in nursing for CAUTI prevention and care of patients with urinary incontinence have evolved to increased collaboration with infection prevention, RN-driven protocols, initiation and continuation of nursing education, and recognition of the part that nursing plays in patient outcomes. The increase in mortality that occurs with CAUTI can be prevented by adhering to evidence-based measures. These measures include appropriate indications for use of indwelling urinary catheters with aseptic technique on insertion, the use of bundles, identification of factors contributing to the patient's urinary incontinence, and use of external urinary collection devices that are correctly applied and managed.

CLINICS CARE POINTS

- Indwelling urinary catheter care:
  - Sterile insertion of the device with 2 nurses present
  - Sterile seal between the catheter and the drainage bag being intact
  - Foley care every 12 hours
  - Make sure the bag never gets two-thirds full, emptying the bag frequently
  - Make sure the bag never touches the floor
  - Use the attached clips to prevent dependent loops in the Foley
  - State lock device must be in place on the inner thigh such that the catheter is not pulling on the urethra
  - Daily assessment of necessity by RN-driven Foley removal protocol

- PureWick:
  - Change device, tubing, and canister every 12 hours or sooner if needed
  - Perform skin check with each device change
  - Suction settings should be intermediate to avoid pressure injury
  - If patient has bowel movement and stool gets on the PureWick, it should be changed
- Condom catheter:
  - Use the correct size catheter each time
  - Use appropriate adhesive and insure the condom catheter is firmly in place with each application
  - Change the condom catheter daily, and the drainage bag as needed
  - Perform skin checks with condom catheter change, looking for edema, skin breakdown, skin tears, and pressure injury

ACKNOWLEDGMENTS

The authors would like to acknowledge Duke Raleigh Hospital Critical Care Medicine, Duke Raleigh Hospital Intensive Care Unit nursing staff for their contributions, with special thanks to critical care nurse Sarah O'Neal, RN.

DISCLOSURE

The authors have nothing to disclose.

REFERENCES

1. Peng D, Li X, Liu P, et al. Epidemiology of pathogens and antimicrobial resistance of catheter-associated urinary tract infections in intensive care units: a systematic review and meta-analysis. Am J Infect Control 2018;46(12):e81–90.
2. Tamadonfar KO, Omattage NS, Spaulding CN, et al. Reaching the end of the line: urinary tract infections. Bact Intracellularity 2019;7(3):83–99.
3. Weiner-Lastinger LM, Abner S, Edwards JR, et al. Antimicrobial-resistant pathogens associated with adult healthcare-associated infections: summary of data reported to the National Healthcare Safety Network, 2015–2017. Infect Control Hosp Epidemiol 2020;41(1):1–18.
4. Hines S. Strengthening national efforts to reduce healthcare-associated infections. AHRQ. 2014. Available at: https://www.ahrq.gov/hai/patient-safety-resources/advances-in-hai/hai-article2.html. Accessed November 30, 2020.
5. Andrade VLF, Fernandes FAV. Prevention of catheter-associated urinary tract infection: implementation strategies of international guidelines. Rev Lat Am Enfermagem 2016;24:e2678.
6. CAUTI guidelines. Centers for Disease Control and Prevention. Available at: https://www.cdc.gov/infectioncontrol/guidelines/cauti/index.html. Accessed November 29, 2020.
7. Jones L, Meyrick J, Bath J, et al. Effectiveness of behavioural interventions to reduce urinary tract infections and Escherichia coli bacteraemia for older adults across all care settings: a systematic review. J Hosp Infect 2019;102(2):200–18.
8. Chenoweth CE, Gould CV, Saint S. Diagnosis, management, and prevention of catheter-associated urinary tract infections. Infect Dis Clin North Am 2014;28(1):105–19.
9. Fasugba O, Koerner J, Mitchell B, et al. Systematic review and meta-analysis of the effectiveness of antiseptic agents for meatal cleaning in the prevention of catheter-associated urinary tract infections. J Hosp Infect 2017;95(3):233–42.

10. Frost SA, Alogso M-C, Metcalfe L, et al. Chlorhexidine bathing and health care-associated infections among adult intensive care patients: a systematic review and meta-analysis. Crit Care 2016;20(1):379.
11. Gould D, Gaze S, Drey N, et al. Implementing clinical guidelines to prevent catheter-associated urinary tract infections and improve catheter care in nursing homes: systematic review. Am J Infect Control 2017;45(5):471–6.
12. Gyesi-Appiah E, Brown J, Clifton A. Short-term urinary catheters and their risks: an integrated systematic review. Br J Nurs 2020;29(9):S16–22.
13. Lord AS, Nicholson J, Lewis A. Infection prevention in the neurointensive care unit: a systematic review. Neurocrit Care 2018;31(1):196–210.
14. Atkins L, Sallis A, Chadborn T, et al. Reducing catheter-associated urinary tract infections: a systematic review of barriers and facilitators and strategic behavioural analysis of interventions. Implement Sci 2020;15(1):44.
15. Hollenbeak CS, Schilling AL. The attributable cost of catheter-associated urinary tract infections in the United States: a systematic review. Am J Infect Control 2018;46(7):751–7.
16. Adams T, Ahnberg M, Alden E, et al. Incontinence device application, male. In: Lippincott nursing procedures. Philadelphia: Wolters Kluwer; 2019. p. 380–2.
17. Mundle W, Howell-Belle C, Jeffs L. Preventing catheter-associated urinary tract infection. J Nurs Care Qual 2020;35(1):83–7.
18. Urinary tract infection (catheter-associated urinary tract infection [CAUTI] and non-catheter-associated urinary tract infection [UTI]) events. National Healthcare Safety Network, Centers for Disease Control and Prevention; 2021. Available at: https://www.cdc.gov/nhsn/pdfs/pscmanual/7psccauticurrent.pdf. Accessed January 1, 2021.
19. Manojlovich M, Lee S, Lauseng D. A systematic review of the unintended consequences of clinical interventions to reduce adverse outcomes. J Patient Saf 2016; 12(4):173–9.
20. Patel PK, Gupta A, Vaughn VM, et al. Review of strategies to reduce central line-associated bloodstream infection (CLABSI) and catheter-associated urinary tract infection (CAUTI) in adult ICUs. J Hosp Med 2017;13(2):105–16.
21. Schreiber PW, Sax H, Wolfensberger A, et al. The preventable proportion of healthcare-associated infections 2005–2016: systematic review and meta-analysis. Infect Control Hosp Epidemiol 2018;39(11):1277–95.
22. Syan R, Brucker BM. Guideline of guidelines: urinary incontinence. BJU Int 2016; 117(1):20–33.
23. Cooper FP, Alexander CE, Sinha S, et al. Policies for replacing long-term indwelling urinary catheters in adults. Cochrane Database Syst Rev 2016;7(7): CD011115.
24. Gray M, Skinner C, Kaler W. External collection devices as an alternative to the indwelling urinary catheter. J Wound Ostomy Continence Nurs 2016;43(3):301–7.

Recruitment and Retention of Minority High School Students to Increase Diversity in the Nursing Profession

Denise Dawkins, DNP, RN, CNL, CHSE

KEYWORDS

- Prenursing students • Black • High school student • Diversity • Underserved
- Culturally competent

KEY POINTS

- Culturally competent health care for minority populations is critical to reducing disparities in health outcomes.
- Increasing diversity in the health workforce will improve the health of unrepresentative populations, as well as the nation.
- Recruitment of Black/African American high school students can create a pipeline of potential culturally competent nursing students.
- Underrepresented students benefit from both emotional and tangible support.
- Appropriate, sound, and successful recruitment strategies require assessment of, and implementing solutions to, challenges.

INTRODUCTION

Disparities in the quality of health care for the Black population have been apparent for many decades,[1,2] evidenced by the high mortality and morbidity rates for the Black/African American community.[3] Major health care organizations have recognized that a culturally diverse nursing workforce is essential to improve the health of this community.[3–5] Recruitment of prenursing students from the Black population is vital to building a diversified workforce sensitive to the community's needs. In recent years, innovative projects have evolved to increase the nurse workforce's diversity by recruiting Black/African American students.[6] This article will provide background, identify challenges, recommend solutions, and showcase successful programs.

The Valley Foundation School of Nursing, San Jose State University, One Washington Square, San Jose, CA 95112, USA
E-mail address: denisedawkins04@gmail.com

Nurs Clin N Am 56 (2021) 427–439
https://doi.org/10.1016/j.cnur.2021.04.007
0029-6465/21/© 2021 The Author. Published by Elsevier Inc. This is an open access article under the
nursing.theclinics.com

BACKGROUND
The Need for a Diverse Workforce to Address Disparities in Health Care

Health disparities in the Black community are reflected in high uninsured rates, high rates of chronic conditions, the highest mortality rate for all cancers combined compared with any other ethnic group, twice the infant death rate than the national average, and poor access to mental health care.[6] One of the factors contributing to these disparities is the lack of culturally competent care, which can lead to unmet health needs and delays in receiving appropriate care.

Although population in the United States is becoming more diverse, this diversity is not reflected in health care or the nurse workforce. The consequences of limited ethnic diversity in the health workforce include increased risk of patient mistrust, segregation, and persistent racial discrimination for some minority groups, including Black/African Americans.[1,7] Ensuring inclusion of Black/African American health care workers in organizations that provide health care in the underserved communities improves access to health care because minorities are often more comfortable with providers of similar racial backgrounds. Minority patients might seek health care sooner if the nurse providing the care were from the same ethnic background.[5]

There is a pressing need to increase the diversity of the nursing workforce as an integral component of efforts to reduce health care disparities due and improve culturally competent care.[1–6] The 2017 survey conducted by the National Council of the State Board of Nursing and the Forum of State Nursing Workforce Center documented the racial/ethnic backgrounds of the registered nurse (RN) population, which was composed of 80.8% white/Caucasian, 6.2% African American, 7.5% Asian, 5.3% Hispanic, 0.4% American Indian/Alaskan Native, 0.5 Native Hawaiian/Pacific Islander, 1.7% two or more races, and 2.9% other nurses.[4] The Black/African American RN population is underrepresented compared with the general minority population of 13% in the United States.[8] One solution to address health inequities would be to increase the number of minority RNs in the health workforce.[3–6]

An effective strategy to increase representation of Black/African nurses in the workforce would be to increase the enrollment of Black/African American high school students in nursing schools.[6] According to National Center for Health Workforce,[5] it is essential to recruit students who live in underserved areas. Active recruitment of underserved high school students can create interest in nursing as a career choice and foster a pipeline of nurses from different backgrounds to enhance the workforce for years to come.

Concurrent with recruitment efforts, strategies for retention are also critical. Retention is important because Black students are at a higher risk for attrition than white nursing students.[9] Black/African American students are essential because they are more likely to stay and serve in the community after graduation.[10,11] Recruitment and retention of this overlooked pool of potential nurses is important to continuing efforts to follow the Institute of Medicine recommendations to increase workforce diversity.[3–6]

Black/African American Nurses in the Workforce

Black/African American nurses in the workforce often understand the inequities that are faced by Black patients and communities.[11] Nurses from underserved communities live in the community spaces and understand the culture from the lens of the population, such as language, values, and shared belief systems. Black/African American nurses can draw from their own experiences and knowledge of the community and are often able to understand the concerns and cultural perspectives of the patient or family members. Black/African American communities are diverse; members may identify as Black, African American, Afro-Latinx, Afro-Brazilian, Afro-Indigenous,

Caribbean, and ethnically of African countries of origin, or otherwise identify with the global African diaspora. Black/African nurses come from these diverse backgrounds and are often about to bring understanding of the perspectives and experiences of the various groups. These nurses can help promote evidence-based care that ensures that these populations receive optimal, empathic, informative, and quality care, enhancing patient outcomes.[5–7,11]

In addition to connecting with underserved patients, nurses from these communities can foster increased trust, challenge institutional biases, and implement strategies that could change health care institutional practice.[12,13] The Black populace has trust issues with the medical community given historical experiences with health care services and health research, such as the Tuskegee syphilis study, men not treated for syphilis, undertreatment of pain, and misappropriation of Henrietta Lacks' cells for research without consent.[14] A quality patient-provider relationship requires trust[7,11] and a cultural connection that may help vulnerable patients feel more comfortable discussing their health concerns.

Barriers to Recruitment and Retention: Connections to Social Determinants of Health Model

The Social Determinants of Health model recognizes that the environmental conditions where people live affect the quality of life and health outcomes.[2,5] Disparities in health are determined, in large part, by these conditions. One of the key domains of social determinants of health involves access to health care services, including consideration of social and cultural barriers to effective care.[2,9,15] Although recruiting diverse health care providers is an important element of improving health care services, barriers to recruitment and retention must be overcome. Many of these barriers are linked to other domains of the social determinants of health model. Social and community contexts (such as discrimination), limited access to enrollment in higher education, and issues with economic stability (eg, poverty) are also key social determinants of health. These conditions, which negatively impact the health of marginalized communities, also create barriers to increasing the diversity in the RN workforce. Consequently, diversifying the nursing workforce requires addressing some of the elements of the Social Determinants of Health model.[16]

Financial instability

Students need income to meet the cost of living, and fees needed to attend high school or college program.[9] High school students could be provided with transportation or resources to cover incidental costs to attend a recruitment program, such as transportation for field trips. Precollege and college selection activities have several incidental costs. Students need funding to cover the cost of applying to college, which includes college admission applications, precollege placement test, and travel cost to visit colleges. Once the student attends college there are tuition, housing, food, transportation, health insurance, incidental fees, and other personal fees.[9]

Education inequality, access, and bias

Black children are less likely to have equal access to quality education opportunities.[17] Some Black children not only have limited access to quality education but also do not have the tools or encouragement to be competitive when applying to nursing school.[17] Some of these children live in neighborhoods with poor-performing schools.[17,18] In addition, Black high school students endure various forms of stereotypes, discrimination, and bias. Some students are exposed to messages that they are not smart enough; they are also less likely to be placed in gifted programs and more likely to be directed to vocational schools.[18,19] Some are labeled as troublemakers and receive unjust punishment.[20] Stereotyping, discrimination, and bias undermine adequate academic preparation for the rigor of nursing school that impacts recruitment of Black students. Students who lack the preparation for college-level courses may not have the grades to qualify for nursing school. For example, poor training in mathematics and science courses and lack of college-level reading, writing, and communication classes can impede access to nursing school.[9] Black students may not be aware of the type and number of required courses in science, math, and English that they must complete at the high school level. In college, freshman and sophomore nursing students have the highest attrition rates due to failure in required science courses.[9] The dropout rate is likely higher among students with inadequate preparation because of substandard education.

Community and social context: shortage of mentors/role models
Black/African American students are bombarded with images of sports figures, musical artist, and acting celebrities as role model representations of viable career options. These glamorous role models may make nursing look less appalling. The nursing profession is often misrepresented in the media with negative images, depicting nurses as uncaring, predominantly white women, or in a way that reinforces stereotypes of female subservience caregivers.[21–23] Throughout history, nurses have been portrayed as white, an angel of mercy, a hero, sex object, shrew, unfeeling, harsh, and the doctor's handmaiden.[23] In addition, the stereotypical image of male nurses depicts "boy toy" gay or medical school dropouts.[24] Professional nurses need to counteract the poor or misleading images, especially of Black/African American nurses, to encourage recruitment of both males and female underrepresented students.

EVIDENCE-BASED SOLUTIONS

It is essential to use evidence-based solutions to reduce barriers and increase recruitment of prospective students from underserved Black communities. Recruitment initiatives should demonstrate sensitivity to diverse stakeholders, including students, families, educators, community organizations, and community leaders. Essential strategies should be inclusive, so students and the community feel respected and valued and trust the program's commitment to student success and community health.[3] The strategies discussed in the following sections have identified some ways to overcome the challenges faced by underrepresented students.

Mentorship and Role Models Matters

Suitable mentors foster nurturing relationships and demonstrate positive characteristics that can reduce the negative impacts of stereotyping, discrimination, and bias.[19] The mentors can enhance social interaction and decrease isolation. Research has shown that mentorship is fundamental because it empowers students, promotes engagement, and helps shape the student's trajectory toward nursing as a career.[19] Mentors often foster an inclusive environment where students can feel supported, respected, and able to have their needs met. Creating a nurturing, safe place for students to overcome expectations of bias and create a sense of belonging can increase Black students' recruitment and retention in nursing.[19]

Black nurses have an important role as mentors and role models who impact others, promote change, and exhibit responsibility, accountability, honesty, and professional integrity for the student nurse population and minority community.[6,9,10,14,19,25] As mentors, Black nurses can demonstrate cultural sensitivity, understand concepts of cultural diversity in health care, and bridge the connection for minority students into the nursing profession.[9,19,26] Black nurse mentors can give students a sense of belonging and often have first-hand experience of a Black student's challenges.[9,19,26] As mentors, they can be effective recruiters and can provide one-one support not only to the student but also to the student's family.[19,26] These nurses, who are working professionals, can provide students with the appropriate intellectual stimulation, challenge, and academic rigor to create meaningful learning opportunities.[6,22,27]

Peer mentors are just as important as a professional mentor because students can identify with them and there are fewer power differences in their relationship as mentor and mentee.[27] Peer mentors, who may look like the student or come from the students' community, are often able to engage in respectful conversation, understand student concerns (eg, socioeconomic challenges or safety issues), and have the student feel valued as prenursing/nursing student. Peer mentors can help socialize the student to the prenursing environment so that students can be successful.[10,26] Another advantage is that some mentors can double as role models.

Role Models

Role models are different from mentors because they serve as an example who can be emulated by students. Ideally, they should inspire students and demonstrate the ability to overcome obstacles; as such it may be helpful for mentors to resemble the student's physical attributes or share other characteristics so they can visually see themselves in the nursing role. This strategy can help the student relate, enhance student confidence and self-efficacy, and excite them about the possibilities.[28] Role models illustrate the process of personal and professional development because they exemplify commitment, good decision making, and how to overcome obstacles. Role models can motivate the student with their stories on how they make it in nursing and navigate through the challenges.[27,28] Mentors are teachers, but accomplished role models can go beyond teaching by modeling skills and behaviors and presenting a positive image of nursing[28,29]

Good role models are a critical component of successful recruitment because students can see the possibilities of becoming a nurse. Black/African American nurses can empower the student by role modeling, setting standards, leading by example, and exhibiting a personal drive to succeed.[25–29] Role models not only demonstrate personal and professional success but also can help counteract the poor or inconsistent images, especially for male nurses.[28,29] For example, one study documented that male African American counselors view nurses as the lowest profession and 1 in 3 counselors admitted not knowing much about nursing.[27] An excellent example of a contemporary role model is Ernest Grant, PhD, RN, the 36th president of the American Nurses Association, the nation's largest nurses' organization, and an African American male. Dr Grant was the youngest of 7 to a single mother and started his nursing career as a licensed practical nurse.[29] Suitable role models and strategic partnerships can enhance a recruitment and retention program.

The Power of Partnerships

Collaboration with partners from a variety of community organization, academic institutions, and professional and social groups can strengthen the recruitment effort.[26,30,31] Community organizations include the neighborhood school, community church, health care facilities, and higher education institutions. The neighborhood church is embedded in the community, well-positioned to improve the congregation's health,[32] and may be committed to recruitment students into nursing. Academic institutions with nursing schools have nurse mentors and role models, peer mentors, and financial resources that may be leveraged for recruitment. Nursing social and professional organizations can supply mentors, role models, and financial resources.[12,19,26,28] Health care facilities can provide financial support and professional mentors/role models. Good collaborations can help reach more students in a recruitment and retention program.[31]

Relationships with organizations like Black sororities and fraternities are important for recruitment. These Black professional organizations were founded on Black college campus and have expanded to other higher colleges and universities. In addition to their commitment to the community, they support educational advancement and enhance social bonds of Black students. The membership includes health and allied professionals who are ideal role models and mentors.[26,28] Another group to enlist in recruitment and retention of students is Black nurses' associations. Such organizations can provide mentors and role models, provide funding resources scholarships, demonstrate professional behavior, and provide a positive nursing image.[2,3,26,28]

Nearby universities and colleges are essential to the recruitment and retention of Black students. Academic institutions have several resources; they have countless mentors and role models, some from the college's nursing department and other health care-related disciplines. Most academic schools have a community service or service leaning requirement for graduation, and college students can make good peer mentors, role models, and emissaries who are culturally sensitive.[22,27] Academic institutions can provide funding and funding collaborations, such as grants and scholarships. Students often need help with applying to college, as it may be difficult to understand the admission process and the postsecondary requirements.[9,19] Other services colleges and universities provide are academic reinforcement; support programs, such as counseling services; tutorials programs, which can improve academic performance; and retention of Black students.[19,25]

The first and most important partnership is with the students' parents or caregivers. Parents' permission is required for activities for high school students. Parents support the student at home regardless of whether the student is in high school or in college. Parents have the inside track to the student that can motivate and support the student.[25,27] It may be helpful to offer a question-and-answer session so that parents can voice their concerns. The best evidence-based program will only be successful if the parent is on board.

Economic and Financial Resources

Financial resources are needed to build capacity, financial assistance for the students, infrastructures such as personal, data collection, marketing, and program evaluation.[9,22,27,33] Successful recruitment and retention programs have sustainable financial support from multiple sources for multiple costs. The Robert Woods Foundation, Occupational Safety and Health Administration, Nurse Workforce Development grants, and Bureau of Health Workforce are committed to improve health care. Effective programs tap into private foundations, professional organizations like nursing organizations/associations, education organizations, sororities and fraternities, community businesses, and colleges and universities for financial support. Some programs receive financial support from in-kind donations,[34] which will help with expenses like books, application fees, tuition, living expenses, and transportation.

Transportation is an important consideration for recruitment programs, and students need financial support for transportation.[25] Students have varying schedules and extracurricular activities and may require reliable transportation to attend meetings or field trips. Scheduling meetings during school time regularly could help attend and eliminate the need for transportation and encourage attendance.[25] When attending college, they need transportation to the college and clinical sites out of school. Maybe a bus transportation company would volunteer the use of their buses for field trips or offer bus passes.[25]

Other financial support students need that could enhance student engagement and retention is funding for college.[9,26,33] The cost of college should not stop a student from attending nursing school. There are financial aids and scholarships available, but sometimes it takes knowledge of where to look. Workshops should be set up for both students and parents to help identify potential sources of funding. Mentor, especially peer mentors, may have experience with funding issues. Students should learn about where to apply for financial aid and scholarships, as well as application deadlines.[9] In addition to learning where and when to apply for funding, students need to learn how to write competitive applications, such as how to play up their strengths, write an outstanding essay, pay attention to details (formatting letters), and look for early options.[9]

Rethink College Admissions Criteria

Holistic admission should be considered to improve recruitment of Black nursing students. Holistic admission is an evidence-based collage admission process that determines the student's eligibility from a wide-ranging criterion.[35,36] The evidence used for admission standard ascertains the students' transcripts, resume, grade point average, college entrance exams, essays, resume, letter of recommendation, and interviews. The admission reviewers are trained about implicit bias, use a descriptive rubric, and sometimes do a blind analysis of the student's records.[35,36] A good example of holistic preadmittance process involves review of the subjective evidence, interviews, essays, or recommendations before the college entrance examination or grade point average. This procedure helps universities holistically, with minimal bias to access the applicant's academic readiness and potential for success in school.[35,36] Some universities use a holistic admission process to use a more equitable process to select a diverse class of students with the background, qualities, and skills needed for success in nursing and support retention of Black students.[35,36]

Putting It All Together: Lessons Learned

Lessons learned from other programs offer valuable guidance for creating or refining recruitment initiatives. In addition to learning from successful programs, it can be just as important to learn from unsuccessful programs with good intentions that failed.[37] Some programs that address social issues fail due to ignorance and arrogance, thinking they know best for the community.[34] Robert Wood Johnson Foundation[37] documented a list of 3 primary reasons for failed social programs: flawed strategy and design, difficult environmental context, and faulty execution.[37] A good example was The Health Professional Partnership Initiative, a program to prepare minority college students for medical school by grooming underrepresented minority elementary and high school students to encourage health careers.[37] The program did not meet expectations and was unable to identify the outcomes of the students. Failure was due to unconnected interventions, lack of knowledge about the large public school system, inability to form effective collaborations, stereotyping/unconscious bias, and inadequate funding.[37] Black communities sometimes resent programmatic decision making and having others presume what they need.[37] The program creators did not understand the culture of community or school system; a mutually beneficial relationship will have openness and flexibility to fix problems that may arise. It can be valuable to review and visit successful programs to learn why they succeeded in order not to make the same mistakes.

Recruiting Black/African American high school students into nursing programs requires a multifaceted and systematic approach. Although there are a range of potential strategies, a successful program design depends on the community's needs and

Table 1
Successful programs for recruiting diverse high school students into the workforce

Program	Key Elements	Key Outcomes
High School Mentoring Program	A national program with a structured case-based curriculum that introduces undeserved high schools to health care careers[34] Targets underserved students[34] Partners and network with local health care/academic facilities[34] Uses stakeholders (volunteers) from the health care community to improve high school education and encourage students to think of college (health care occupations) as a viable option[34]	Student alumni become role models for their community Students consider health care careers after exposure to these programs[34] In the California Partnership Academies, graduation rates exceeded state-wide rates, and African American and Latinx seniors had the highest point increase[34]
Project BEST (Black Excellence in Scholarship and Teaching)	Partnerships between the community, the area high schools, local university, business community, parents, and student[38] Mentorship Focus on high school Black males Start freshman year Assist with college preparatory activities (college applications, SAT/ACT, and scholarships)[38]	Award scholarships Provides mentors and role models Follow-up with students after college[38]
Summer internship programs	Addressing the nursing shortage by recruiting potential minority nursing student to pursue a nursing career[27,33] Classroom activities, field trips, hospital tours[27] Structured activities, mathematics, reading, health and science, and social skills activities[33] Occurs during off-school sessions	Students surveyed had a strong desire to become a registered nurse[27,33] Broaden students' concept of what constitutes health care career, career attainable, and intrinsic rewarding[35]

(*continued on next page*)

Table 1 (continued)		
Program	**Key Elements**	**Key Outcomes**
Nurse/Medical Explorers Sponsored by Boy Scouts of America or hospitals	High schools are exposed to health care careers to encourage medical careers. Activities include regular meetings and activities with parent involvement[39]	Medical Explorer Post 4077, Texas University: established since 1991. Successful health care provider graduates return to mentors' new members[39]
Virtual[40]	Foster unrepresentative students interested in health care careers Focus on urban youth Hands-on experience and access to positive role models Use e-learning, pod cast, virtual webinars[40]	More students were able to attend due to the virtual platform, no interference with their schedule One program documented that 87% who apply to medical school were accepted. MCAT scores increased by 8–10 points[40]
Bureau of Health Workforce	Adopted the transformation from health disparities to health equity model[4] Incorporates concept of social determinants as a framework to facilitate nursing workforce[4] Implemented holistic admission[4] Used framework social determines as funding opportunities[4]	More than 92 schools of nursing received awards that used the framework[4] 2014–2015: 4444 students trained from underserved minorities or disadvantaged background[4]
Nursing school programs	A comprehensive year-round preentry baccalaureate preparation program, targeting high school students from disadvantaged backgrounds Multidiscipline team, RN, social worker, & case manager Structure math & science curriculum Summer activity: certified nursing aid training Seniors admitted to university[41]	Graduation rate 85% First time NCLEX 100% 82% found employment after graduation Some continued their education[41]

(continued on next page)

Table 1 (continued)		
Program	**Key Elements**	**Key Outcomes**
Retention nursing programs	Training program to support nursing students (2008–2015)[12] Underrepresented/ underserved racial and ethnic groups[12] Students receive financial, academic, social/ emotional/cultural, and leadership and professional support year round[28] Funded by Robert Woods Foundation and AACN's NCIN scholarship program with health career-oriented educational interventions. Grants went out to 130 schools[42]	65% earn BSN GPA & NCLEX scores improved, 70% graduated[12] 2706 individuals earned the BSN degree and 801 earned their master's Meeting nursing demand through diversity[42]

Abbreviations: AACN, American Association of College of Nursing; ACT, American College Test; BSN, Bachelor of Nursing; GPA, Grade point Average; MCAT, Medical College Admission Test; NCIN, New Careers in Nursing; NCLX, National Council Licensure Examination; RN, registered nurse; SAT, Scholastic Aptitude Test.

resources. For example, programs may have different methods and vary in length, partnerships, and services. **Table 1** summarizes the elements and the outcomes of several successful programs.

SUMMARY

Improving the diversity of the RN nursing workforce is important to advancing health equity. Recruitment initiatives can improve Black/African American students' awareness of and desire for nursing as a viable career choice. One way to recruit and retain these potential nurses is to understand the challenges these students face. Some significant challenges students face include bias, lack of mentioning and role models, and financial issues. Students like to belong and feel a part of a group, so emotional and social support should be a high priority. Good leadership and professional development necessitate support, nurturing, and role modeling/mentoring for the student. The student participant should be in a safe environment that promotes engagement and affirmation and recognizes their full potential to pursue nursing as a career. Solutions to overcome these challenges regarding recruiting and retaining diverse underserved students consist of evidence-based interventions. Successful programs prepare students for college and nursing as a career option after college.

CLINICS CARE POINTS

- Advocate for the need to diversify the nurse workforce
- Recognize the need to enhance the enrollment of Black/African American students in nursing school programs

- Understand what social determinants of health model can identify barriers for Black/African American students
  - Financial instability: Students need income to meet the cost of living and school expenses
  - Education inequality: Black children are less likely to have equal access to quality education
  - Black high school students endure various forms of stereotypes, discrimination, and bias
  - Community and social context: Shortage of mentors/role models
- Define goals to enhance enrollment of Black/African American students in nursing schools
- Create a plan using an evidence-based solution

CONFLICT OF INTEREST STATEMENT

The authors declare that the article was conducted in the absence of any commercial or financial relationships that could be construed as a potential conflict of interest.

REFERENCES

1. Baldwin DM. Disparities in health and health care: focusing efforts to eliminate unequal burdens. Online J Issues Nurs 2003;8(1):2. Accessed December 2, 2020.
2. Sondik EJ, Huang DT, Klein RJ, et al. Progress toward the healthy people 2010 goals and objectives. Annu Rev Public Health 2010;31:271–81. https://doi.org/10.1146/annurev.publhealth.012809.103613, 4 p folliwng 281. Accessed December 1, 2020.
3. American Association of Colleges of Nursing. Enhancing diversity in the workforce. American association of colleges of nursing Web site 2015. Available at: http://www.aacn.nche.edu/media-relations/fact-sheets/enhancing-diversity. Accessed December 1, 2020.
4. Spencer TD. Improving diversity of the nursing workforce through evidence-based strategies. J Nurs Educ 2020;59(7):363–4.
5. Office of Disease and Health Promotion. Health people 2020: social determinants of health. 2020. Available at: https://www.healthypeople.gov/2020/topics-objectives/topic/Access-to-Health-Services. Accessed December 1, 2020.
6. Sullivan LW. Missing persons: minorities in the health professions, A report of the Sullivan commission on diversity in the healthcare workforce. 2004. Available at: https://search.datacite.org/works/10.13016/cwij-acxl. Accessed December 1, 2020.
7. Schantz S, Charron SA, Folden SL. Health seeking behaviors of Haitian families for their school aged children. J Cult Divers 2003;10(2):62–8. Available at: https://www.ncbi.nlm.nih.gov/pubmed/14508927. Accessed December 1, 2020.
8. Black population: 2010. 2010 census brief: Census briefs;2011 ASI 2326-17.201; census C2010BR-06 2011. Accessed December 1, 2020.
9. Nnedu CC. Recruiting and retaining minorities in nursing education. ABNF J 2009;20(4):93–6. Available at: https://www.ncbi.nlm.nih.gov/pubmed/19927893. Accessed December 12, 2020.
10. Elfman L. Meeting Nursing Demand Through Diversity. Diverse issues in higher education February 25, 201. December 2020. Available at: https://diverseeducation.com/article/110965/. Accessed December 1, 2020.
11. Sullivan LS. Trust, risk, and race in american medicine. Hastings Cent Rep 2020;50(1):18–26. Available at: https://onlinelibrary.wiley.com/doi/abs/10.1002/hast.1080.

12. Nursing workforce projections by ethnicity and race, 2014-2030: National center for health workforce analysis reports;2018 ASI 4116-11.50.2018. December 2020. Available at: https://statistical.proquest.com/statisticalinsight/result/pqpresultpage.previewtitle?docType=PQSI&titleUri=/content/2018/4116-11.50.xml. Accessed December 1, 2020.

13. Wenfield Adia. The disproportionate impact of covid-19 on Black health care workers in the U.S. Harvard Business Review Home. 2020. 2020. Available at: https://hbr.org/2020/05/the-disproportionate-impact-of-covid-19-on-Black-health-care-workers-in-the-u-s.

14. Washington HA. Medical apartheid the dark history of medical experimentation on Black Americans from colonial times to the present. New York: Random House Inc; 2006.

15. Office of disease and health promotion. Health people social determinants of health. U.S. Department of health and human services Web site. 2020. Available at: https://www.healthypeople.gov/2020/topics-objectives/topic/social-determinants-of-health. Accessed December 12, 2020.

16. Solar O, Irwin A. A conceptual framework for action on the social determinants of health (paper 2)2007. Available at: http://health-equity.pitt.edu/757. Accessed December 12, 2020.

17. Office of Disease and Health Promotion. Healthy people 2030; education access and quality. U.S. Department of Health and Human Services. Available at: https://health.gov/healthypeople/objectives-and-data/browse-objectives/education-access-and-quality. Accessed December 14, 2020.

18. Walker EN. Why Aren't more minorities taking advanced Math? Education Leadership. November 2 65 (3) Making Math Count Pages 48-53. Available at: http://www.ascd.org/publications/educational-leadership/nov07/vol65/num03/Why-Aren%2527t-More-Minorities-Taking-Advanced-Math%25C2%25A2.aspx. Accessed November 20, 2020.

19. Holden L, Rumala B, Carson P, et al. Promoting careers in health care for urban youth: What students, parents and educators. Can Teach Us 2014;34(3–4):355–66. Accessed November 20, 2020.

20. American Psychological Association. Inequality at school What's behind the racial disparity in our education system?. Available at: https://www.apa.org/monitor/2016/11/cover-inequality-school 2020. Accessed November 20, 2020.

21. Whelan J. Does American nursing have A diversity problem? 2015University of Pennsylvania School of Nursing. Available at: https://historian.nursing.upenn.edu/2015/02/26/diversity_nursing/. Accessed November 20, 2020.

22. Godsey JA, Houghton DM, Hayes T. Registered nurse perceptions of factors contributing to the inconsistent brand image of the nursing profession. Nurs Outlook 2020;68(6):808–21.

23. Anthony M, Turner JA, Novell M. (May 31, 2019) "Fiction Versus Reality: Nursing Image as Portrayed by Nursing Career Novels" OJIN: The Online 24, (2), Manuscript 4. Available at: https://ojin.nursingworld.org/MainMenuCategories/ANAMarketplace/ANAPeriodicals/OJIN/TableofContents/Vol-24-2019/No2-May-2019/Fiction-vs-Reality-Nursing-Image.html. Accessed November 20, 2020.

24. Patino Erica. Lights, Camera, Accuracy: Nurses in the Media. *Minority Nurse*. Available at: https://minoritynurse.com/lights-camera-accuracy-nurses-in-the-media/. Accessed November 20, 2020.

25. Woods-Giscombe CL, Rowsey PJ, Kneipp S, et al. Student perspective on recruiting underrepresented ethnic minority students to nursing: Enhancing

outreach, engaging family, and correcting misconceptions. J Prof Nurs 2020; 36(Issue 2):43–9.

26. Phillip JM, Malone B. Increasing racial/ethnic diversity in nursing to reduce health disparities and achieve health equity. Public Health Rep 2014;(supp):40–50. https://doi.org/10.1177/00333549141291S209.

27. Matutina RE. Recruiting Middle School Students into Nursing. J Sch Nurs 2008; 24:11–115.

28. Diefenbeck CA, Klemm PR. Outcomes of a workforce diversity retention program for underrepresented minority and disadvantaged students in a baccalaureate nursing program. J Prof Nurs 2020. https://doi.org/10.1016/j.profnurs.2020.06.001.

29. Nelson R. Ernest Grant Breaks Barriers. Am J Nurs 2019;119(1):65–6. Available at: http://ovidsp.ovid.com/ovidweb.cgi?T=JS&NEWS=n&CSC=Y&PAGE=fulltext&D= ovft&AN=00000446-201901000-00035. Accessed November 20, 2020.

30. Bianco M, Leech N, Mitchell k. Pathways to teaching African American male teens explore teaching as a career. J Negro Educ 2011;80(3):368. Available at: http://search.proquest.com.libaccess.sjlibrary.org/docview/9033033 247accountid = 10361. Accessed December 1, 2020.

31. Robert Woods Johnson Foundation. Mentoring to build a culture of health. August 15, 2014. Available at: https://www.rwjf.org/en/blog/2014/08/mentoring_to_ builda.html. Accessed December 1, 2020.

32. Giger JN, Appel SJ, Davidhizar R, et al. Church and spirituality in the lives of the African American community. J Transcult Nurs 2008;19(4):375–83.

33. Condon VM, Morgan CJ, Miller EW, et al. A program to enhance recruitment and retention of disadvantaged and ethnically diverse baccalaureate nursing students. J Transcultural Nurs 2013;24(4):397–407. Available at: https://journals. sagepub.com/doi/full/10.1177/1043659613493437.

34. Dayton C, Hamilton C, Stern H. Profile of the California partnership academies. California Department of Education, with support from the Department and the James Irvine; 2011. Available at: https://www.cde.ca.gov/ci/gs/hs/cpareport09.asp.

35. Grijalva C. Holistic Admissions Recruiting and Admitting Diverse Students. Sacramento, California, December 08, 2020. Webinar.

36. Glazer G, Clark A, Bankston K, et al. Holistic Admissions in Nursing: We Can Do This. J Prof Nurs 2016;32(4):306–13.

37. Isaacs S, Colby D. Good Ideas at the time: Learning from programs that did not work out as expected, Robert Woods Johnson Foundation To improve Health Care, XIII.

38. Project BEST Black Excellence in Scholarship and Teaching. Available at: https:// www.kernhigh.org/apps/pages/project-best. Accessed December 1, 2020.

39. Texas State University. Medical explorer post 4077. 2020. Available at: https:// www.bio.txstate.edu/medicalexplorers/. Accessed December 1, 2020.

40. Fernandez-Repollet E, Locatis C, De Jesus-Monge WE, et al. Effects of summer internship and follow-up distance mentoring programs on middle and high school student perceptions and interest in health careers. BMC Med Educ 2018;18(1): 84. Available at: https://search.datacite.org/works/10.1186/s12909-018-1205-3.

41. Colville J, Cottom S, Robinette T, et al. A community college model to support nursing workforce diversity. J Nurs Educ 2015;54(2):65–71.

42. Robert Woods Johnson Foundation. New Careers in Nursing 2008-2015. December 2020. Available at: http://www.newcareersinnursing.org/. Accessed December 1, 2020.

Nursing Simulation Debriefing: Useful Tools

Michele L. Kuszajewski, DNP, RN, CHSE

KEYWORDS

- Debriefing • Feedback • Facilitation • Guided reflection • Experiential learning
- Simulation-based education

KEY POINTS

- Debriefing is a structured, collaborative, and reflective process following a simulation learning activity.
- A structured debriefing is a vital part of simulation-based education.
- Debriefing should be led by a trained facilitator using evidence-based or theory-based methods.
- The simulation facilitator should receive formal training, ongoing professional development, and evaluation to ensure implementation of debriefing best practices.

INTRODUCTION

Over the past several years, simulation-based education (SBE) has been widely used to train nursing students and other health care professionals. Simulation is an interactive educational technique that mimics real-life events and provides opportunities to promote learning, practice, and/or evaluation in a controlled safe environment.[1(p43),2(pS44)] Simulation is a form of experiential learning that consists of learning by doing, reflecting on the experience and assimilating lessons learned into behaviors.[3,4]

A simulation activity consists of 3 components—prebrief, scenario, and debrief—which are led by a simulation facilitator. The simulation facilitator is a trained educator who delivers the simulation activity and provides guidance, support, and structure to the postevent discussion to enhance learning.[1(p18),2(pS42)] The simulation activity begins with a prebrief. The prebrief is an introduction by the simulation facilitator outlining learner expectations, roles, and responsibilities and orienting the learner to the environment, manikin, and equipment.[2,4] During the prebrief, the facilitator also acknowledges their awareness that the simulation is not real but instead is a technique to replace or mimic real-life experiences. The facilitator assures the learners that this is

Center for Nursing Discovery, Duke University School of Nursing, 307 Trent Drive, DUMC Box 3322, Durham, NC 27710, USA
E-mail address: michele.kuszajewski@duke.edu

Nurs Clin N Am 56 (2021) 441–448
https://doi.org/10.1016/j.cnur.2021.05.003
0029-6465/21/© 2021 Elsevier Inc. All rights reserved.

a safe learning environment to develop or enhance knowledge, skills, and behaviors in a controlled, nonjudgmental manner.[5] Learners are encouraged to immerse themselves into the simulation activity and suspend disbelief. The prebrief sets the foundation for learning and lasts approximately 10 minutes.

The prebrief transitions to the actual simulation experience or delivery of the simulation scenario. The simulation scenario is developed to create an environment or situation close to a clinical event or situation for learning and skills acquisition.[6] The scenario should be delivered in a setting where learners feel safe to participate and engage in the learning process. The length of the simulation scenario depends on the learning objectives but typically last approximately 20 minutes to 30 minutes.

The simulation scenario is followed by a reflective discussion and analysis of the simulation activity to identify and close the gaps in knowledge and skills.[5-7] This discussion, known as the debrief, provides a means for reflection-on-action and reflection-after-action and is key to the experiential learning.[5,7,8] Although each phase of the simulation activity is significant, this article focuses on the final phase of the simulation activity—the debrief.

WHAT IS DEBRIEFING?

Debriefing is defined as a structured, collaborative, and reflective process within the simulation learning activity led by a trained simulation facilitator using an evidenced-based or theory-based debriefing model.[1(p14),2(pS41)] Debriefing is a vital part of SBE where many experts believe a large portion of the learning occurs.[4-8]

So what is the purpose of debriefing in nursing education? Debriefing is a form of feedback where the communication is interactive, bidirectional, and learner-centered.[7,8] This deliberate discussion between the facilitator and learners following a simulation activity provides opportunities for learner reflection. Debriefing includes (1) reexamining the simulation scenario, (2) gaining a clear understanding of thought processes and actions, and (3) promoting learning objectives to enhance learning and change in clinical performance.[4-6,9] Timely feedback is important aspect of SBE and most often is completed immediately following the simulation activity.[4,5,8] Debriefing is an integral part of learner education and integration across the nursing curriculum should be considered for use in the simulation laboratory, classroom, and clinical setting.[10]

PHASES OF DEBRIEFING

Experts have identified 3 common elements or phases of debriefing.[11-15] These include the reaction, understanding/analysis, and summary phases.

1. Reaction phase—this phase is described as emotion before cognition[9] and provides the learner with the opportunity to release emotion and express feelings (affective domain). Learners need time to purge initial emotions to decrease stress they may have experienced during the simulation scenario to move into reflective discussion.[9] Facilitators may begin this discussion by asking the learner, "How did that feel?" or "How are you feeling right now?" This phase typically lasts approximately 5 minutes.
2. Understanding or analysis phase—throughout the simulation activity, the facilitator observes and evaluates the learner's conversation and actions and notes these for the postevent discussion (cognitive domain). The facilitator identifies topics of discussion that are aligned with the learning objectives. During this phase, the facilitator explores the learners thought process during the simulation scenario by

using open-ended questions or Socratic questioning. This type of questioning is useful in assisting learners in identifying and closing the gaps in knowledge and skills. At this point the learners begin to conceptualize how the points discussed are applicable to clinical practice.[9] The facilitator may ask, "What were you thinking when ....?"[6] A majority of the debrief discussion is spent in the understanding or analysis phase.

3. Summary phase—this phase concludes the debrief session. The facilitator makes the learners aware that this is the wrap-up or end phase of the debrief. This phase is grounded in the learning objectives and includes discussion of lessons learned.[5] The facilitator may ask the learners, "Can you share with us something you learned today that you will take to the clinical setting?" or "What is something that went well and something you would like to improve on?" The facilitator uses this time to close the loop on the discussion of the learning objectives and ensure take away points are identified by the learner. This phase typically lasts less than 10 minutes.

DEBRIEFING PRACTICES AND CONSIDERATIONS

An effective debriefing requires training, planning, and purposeful implementation of simulation best practices by the facilitator. As part of SBE best practices, the facilitator considers the environment, ground rules, and communication techniques to meet the learning objectives.[2(pS22)]

The debriefing must take place in an environment or setting where learners feel safe to engage in discussion and reflect on their actions and performance.[2,(pS22),4,5,9] Physical and psychological safety is crucial for learning to occur. When possible, the facilitator should debrief in an area separate from where the simulation scenario occurred and position themselves among learners for this discussion to avoid perception of hierarchy during the discussion.[4] Ensuring psychological safety during the debrief is vital. Learners need assurance that their performance and discussion will remain confidential and not shared with other learners, faculty or staff. The facilitator must provide a supportive climate where learners feel valued, respected and free to learn.[4] These concepts of safety are introduced by the facilitator in the prebrief and reinforced throughout the simulation scenario and again at the beginning of the debrief.

The next important component of the debrief is establishing ground rules and a shared mental model. For a productive debriefing discussion between the facilitator and learners, ground rules, or stated expectations and a shared mental model must be identified. Many facilitators include the Center for Medical Simulation's The Basic Assumption statement in the prebrief and debrief to assist with this process. The Basic Assumption states, "We believe that everyone participating in this simulation is intelligent, well-trained, cares about doing their best, and wants to improve."[16] Ground rules often include the expectation of respectful and active participation in discussion and confidentiality during and after the debrief. Developing a shared mental model or mutual understanding of the ground rules and events that occurred during the simulation scenario also supports reflective discussion.

Clear and effective communication by the facilitator is another consideration during the debrief that contributes to the learning environment. This includes use of open-ended questions, active listening, and appropriate use of nonverbal clues. Use of open-ended questions or cue questions encourages conversation and leads to more extensive learner participation in the debrief. Another communication technique that is important to the facilitator-learner relationship is active listening. During the debrief discussion, the facilitator must be simply listening, not listening for the purpose to respond.[5] During the debrief, silence may occur. The facilitator needs to be comfortable with this silence and give learners time to process their thoughts and emotions before sharing.[4,8] Most educators wait less than 1 second after asking learners a question before answering it themselves.[17] In an effort to promote learner involvement, the facilitator should pose a question and then patiently wait for an answer.

Another communication technique to promote learning is the use of nonverbal cues. During the debrief, the facilitator should display open body language and use good eye contact and show affirmation or reassurance by nodding. Because debriefing is learner-centered, the facilitator should guide and direct the discussion (not lecture) in order for learners to analyze their own performance and actively contribute to their learning.[4] Using effective communication techniques, the facilitator guides the reflective discussion by providing constructive feedback, addressing specific aspects of the learner's performance, and focusing on the learning objectives.[8]

DEBRIEFING METHODS

There are several evidence-based or theory-based methods of debriefing. These include but are not limited to Debriefing with Meaningful Learning (DML); Debriefing with Good Judgment (DGJ); the gather, analyze, and summarize (GAS) model; and Promoting Excellence and Reflective Learning in Simulation (PEARLS). **Table 1** provides tools and strategies to guide the reflection on the learning that occurred during the simulation scenario. The choice of debriefing method should match the simulation activity, learning objectives, facilitator preference, and skill.[5] It is not uncommon for the facilitator to use more than 1 method to debrief.

Table 1
Evidenced based Debriefing Methods

Debriefing Model	Description	Reference
DML	• DML uses 6 phases: engage, explore, explain, elaborate, evaluate, and extend. • DML looks at the reflective process: reflection-in-action, reflection-on-action and reflection-beyond-action. • DML uses Socratic questioning and principles of active learning to uncover learner thinking associated with their actions: who, what, where, when, why, and how? • Facilitator does not readily give information or answers questions. Discussion is learner-directed, where the learner states the answer or becomes aware of their knowledge gaps. • DML is a method of reflective learning that facilitates the development of clinical reasoning.	Dreifuerst KT. The essentials of debriefing in simulation learning: A concept analysis. *Nursing Education Perspectives.* 2009; 30(2):109–114.[11] Dreifuerst KT. Getting started with debriefing for meaningful learning. *Clinical Simulation in Nursing.* 2015; 11(5):268–275.[12]

(continued on next page)

Table 1 (continued)		
Debriefing Model	**Description**	**Reference**
DGJ	• DGJ uses 3 phases: reaction, analysis, and summary. • DGJ uses is a nonjudgmental approach rather than harsh criticism of learner performance. • DGJ focuses on creating a context for adult learners (including the facilitator) to learn important lessons that will help them move toward key objectives. • DJG focuses not only on the learner actions but also on the meaning of the learner's frames, assumptions, and knowledge. • DGJ shares the expert view of the facilitator as a way to initiate discussion with the learner.	Rudolph JW, Simon R, Dufresne RL, Raemer DB. There's No Such Thing as "Nonjudgmental" Debriefing: A Theory and Method for Debriefing with Good Judgment. *Simulation in Healthcare.* 2006; 1(1):49–55.[13] Rudolph JW, Simon R, Rivard P, Dufresne RL, Raemer DB. Debriefing with Good Judgment: Combining Rigorous Feedback with Genuine Inquiry. *Anesthesiology Clinics.* 2007; 25(2):361–376.[18]
GAS model	• GAS uses 3 phases: gather, analyze, and summarize. • Referred to as a structured and supportive debrief model • Gather phase: the facilitator can ask the learners about their observations or share what they observed. This phase is used mostly to gauge learner reaction to simulation and clarify facts about what happened. • Analyze phase: the facilitator asks the "why" behind each learner action in the simulation in attempt to understand their reasoning behind their actions. This phase involves in-depth discussion of observed performance or perception gaps. • Summarize phase: ends the debriefing session with question, such as, "What are the main things you learned about...?" In this phase, the learners verbalize "take away points" or need for performance improvement.	Cheng A, Rodgers DL, Van Der Jagt É, Eppich W, O'Donnell J. Evolution of the Pediatric Advanced Life Support course: enhanced learning with a new debriefing tool and Web-based module for Pediatric Advanced Life Support instructors. *Pediatric Critical Care Medicine.* 2012; 13(5):589–595.[14] Phrampus PE, O'Donnell JM. Debriefing Using a Structured and Supported Approach. In: Levine AI, DeMaria S, Schwartz AD, Sim AJ, eds. *The Comprehensive Textbook of Healthcare Simulation.* Springer New York; 2013:73–84.[6]

(continued on next page)

Table 1 *(continued)*		
Debriefing Model	**Description**	**Reference**
PEARLS	• PEARLS uses 4 phases: reaction, description, analysis, and summary. • PEARLS integrates 3 common educational strategies, including learner self-assessment, facilitating focused discussion, and providing information in the form of directive feedback and/or teaching. • PEARLS incorporates scripted language to guide the debriefing.	Eppich W, Cheng A. Promoting Excellence and Reflective Learning in Simulation (PEARLS): Development and Rationale for a Blended Approach to Health Care Simulation Debriefing. *Simulation in Healthcare.* 2015; 10(2):106–115.[15]

TRAINING TO FACILITATE DEBRIEFING

Debriefing, often described as an art and a science, is a complex skill requiring formal training in the development and maintenance of observational and interviewing skills.[6,9,19–21] The quality of the debrief and impact of learning depend on the skills of the facilitator.[4,6,9,22] To ensure best practices, a facilitator must be trained formally and deemed competent in the theory and delivery of debriefing.[2(pS22),22] This competency requires knowledge of the learning objectives, understanding of the needs of the learner, and skills in guided reflection.

Professional development requires time and financial investment. Researchers found that only 31% of nursing schools use theory-based models to guide debriefing and less than half of all facilitators have had any type of training.[22] Debriefing training can be obtained by educational programs offered by simulation centers, workshops at conferences, or seeking fellowship training or advanced degree in simulation.[19,20] Following initial training practice, mentorship and evaluation are ongoing.[10,19–21]

SUMMARY

Debriefing is a structured, collaborative, and reflective process following a simulation learning activity and is a vital part of SBE. Debriefing is a guided reflective discussion led by a trained facilitator using evidence-based methods. The debriefing is learner-centered and includes bidirectional conversation between the facilitator and learners to identify and close the gaps in knowledge and skills.

The simulation facilitator should receive formal training, ongoing professional development and evaluation to ensure debriefing best practices are applied. There are several theory-based debriefing methods to guide the facilitation. Integration of debriefing into the nursing curriculum and application of debriefing methods in the laboratory, classroom, and clinical settings will elevate a nursing student's learning in assist in closing the gaps in knowledge and performance in each of these settings.

DISCLOSURE

The author has nothing to disclose.

REFERENCES

1. Lioce L, Lopreiato J, Downing D, et al, editors. The terminology and concepts working group (2020), healthcare simulation dictionary –. 2nd Edition. Rockville, MD: Agency for Healthcare Research and Quality; 2020. AHRQ Publication No. 20-0019.
2. INACSL Standards Committee. INACSL standards of best practice: simulation©: simulation. Clin Simulation Nurs 2016;12:S5–50.
3. Kolb DA. Experiential learning: experience as the source of learning and development. Upper Sadle River: Prentice Hall; 1984.
4. Fanning RM, Gaba DM. The role of debriefing in simulation-based learning. Simulation Healthc 2007;2(2):115–25.
5. Bauchat JR, Seropian M. Essentials of debriefing in simulation-based education. In: Comprehensive healthcare simulation: anesthesiology. Cham: Springer; 2020. p. 37–46.
6. Phrampus PE, O'Donnell JM. Debriefing using a structured and supported approach. In: Levine AI, DeMaria S, Schwartz AD, et al, editors. The comprehensive textbook of healthcare simulation. New York: Springer; 2013. p. 73–84.
7. Raemer D, Anderson M, Cheng A, et al. Research regarding debriefing as part of the learning process. Simulation Healthc 2011;6(Suppl):S52–7.
8. Sawyer T, Eppich W, Brett-Fleegler M, et al. More than one way to debrief: a critical review of healthcare simulation debriefing methods. Simulation Healthc 2016; 11(3):209–17.
9. Palaganas JC, Fey M, Simon R. Structured Debriefing in Simulation-Based Education. AACN Adv Crit Care 2016;27(1):78–85.
10. National League for Nursing (NLN). Debriefing across the curriculum: a living document from the national league for nursing 2015. Available at: http://www.nln.org/docs/default-source/about/nln-vision-series-(position-statements)/nln-vision-debriefing-across-the-curriculum.pdf?sfvrsn=0.
11. Dreifuerst KT. The essentials of debriefing in simulation learning: a concept analysis. Nurs Educ Perspect 2009;30(2):109–14.
12. Dreifuerst KT. Getting started with debriefing for meaningful learning. Clin Simulation Nurs 2015;11(5):268–75.
13. Rudolph JW, Simon R, Dufresne RL, et al. There's No Such Thing as "Nonjudgmental" debriefing: a theory and method for debriefing with good judgment. Simulation Healthc 2006;1(1):49–55.
14. Cheng A, Rodgers DL, Van Der Jagt É, et al. Evolution of the pediatric advanced life support course: enhanced learning with a new debriefing tool and web-based module for pediatric advanced life support instructors. Pediatr Crit Care Med 2012;13(5):589–95.
15. Eppich W, Cheng A. Promoting excellence and reflective learning in simulation (PEARLS): development and rationale for a blended approach to health care simulation Debriefing. Simulation Healthc 2015;10(2):106–15.
16. The Center for Medical Simulation. The basic Assumption™. Available at: https://harvardmedsim.org/resources/the-basic-assumption/ (Copyright 2004-2020).
17. Anderson S. Actively involving students in learning: considerations when approaching a new semester. 2011. Available at: https://learninginnovation.duke.edu/blog/2011/10/actively-involving-students/. Accessed December 1, 2020.
18. Rudolph JW, Simon R, Rivard P, et al. Debriefing with good judgment: combining rigorous feedback with genuine inquiry. Anesthesiol Clin 2007;25(2):361–76.

19. Cheng A, Grant V, Huffman J, et al. Coaching the debriefer: peer coaching to improve debriefing quality in simulation programs. Simulation Healthc 2017; 12(5):319–25.

20. Cheng A, Grant V, Dieckmann P, et al. Faculty development for simulation programs: five issues for the future of debriefing training. Simulation Healthc 2015; 10(4):217–22.

21. Dieckmann P, Molin Friis S, Lippert A, et al. The art and science of debriefing in simulation: ideal and practice. Med Teach 2009;31(7):e287–94.

22. Fey MK, Jenkins LS. Debriefing practices in nursing education programs: results from a national study. Nurs Educ Perspect 2015;36(6):361–6.

Moving?

Make sure your subscription moves with you!

To notify us of your new address, find your **Clinics Account Number** (located on your mailing label above your name), and contact customer service at:

Email: journalscustomerservice-usa@elsevier.com

800-654-2452 (subscribers in the U.S. & Canada)
314-447-8871 (subscribers outside of the U.S. & Canada)

Fax number: 314-447-8029

Elsevier Health Sciences Division
Subscription Customer Service
3251 Riverport Lane
Maryland Heights, MO 63043

*To ensure uninterrupted delivery of your subscription, please notify us at least 4 weeks in advance of move.

Printed and bound by CPI Group (UK) Ltd, Croydon, CR0 4YY

03/10/2024

01040467-0013